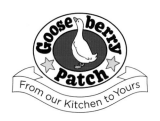

400-Calorie Slow-Cooker Recipes

Delicious and satisfying dishes for every meal, plus desserts and snacks!

To cooks everywhere who want to watch calories and save time by making healthy slow-cooked meals the entire family will enjoy!

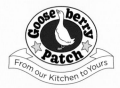

Gooseberry Patch
An imprint of Globe Pequot
246 Goose Lane
Guilford, CT 06437

**www.gooseberrypatch.com
1 800 854 6673**

Copyright 2018, Gooseberry Patch
978-1-62093-267-4

· ·

Do you have a tried & true recipe... tip, craft or memory that you'd like to see featured in a **Gooseberry Patch** cookbook? Visit our website at www. gooseberrypatch.com and follow the easy steps to submit your favorite family recipe.

Or send them to us at:
Gooseberry Patch
PO Box 812
Columbus, OH 43216-0812

Don't forget to include the number of servings your recipe makes, plus your name, address, phone number and email address. If we select your recipe, your name will appear right along with it... and you'll receive a FREE copy of the book!

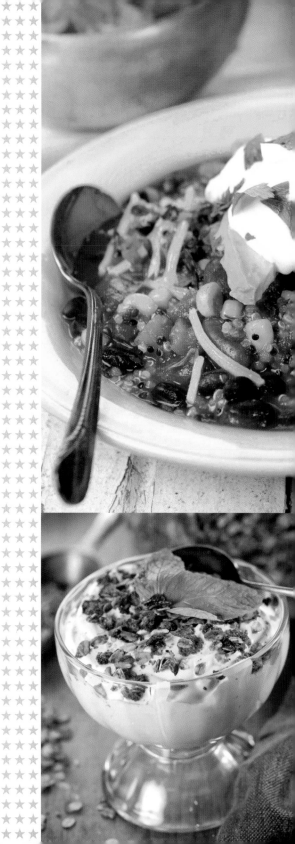

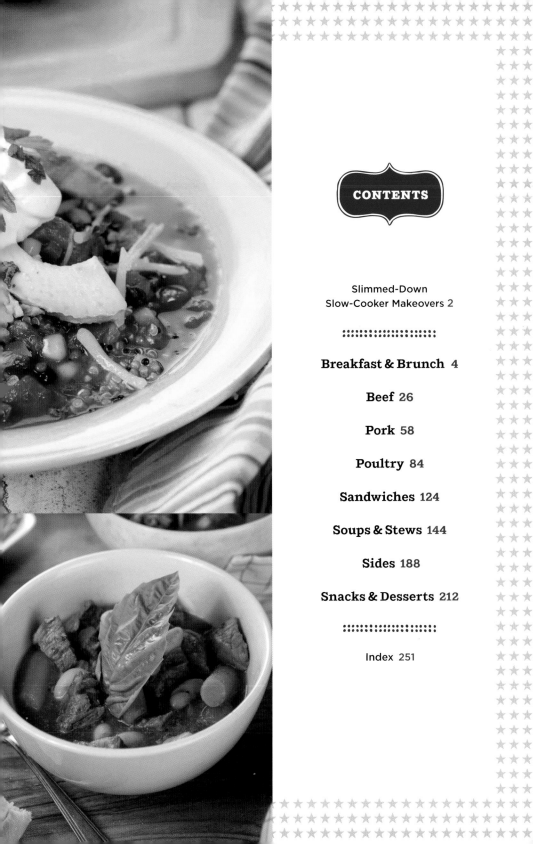

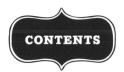
CONTENTS

Slimmed-Down Slow-Cooker Makeovers

Do you crave your favorite slow-cooked dishes, but don't want all the calories from those familiar comfort foods? Well, we've found a way to cut the calories in over 150 family-friendly dishes without sacrificing flavor or decadent deliciousness. Without ruling out any foods, we've kept an eye out for portion control while ensuring each morsel in every downsized dish is incredibly satisfying. Now, you can dive into the foods you love...and feel good in doing so.

With smart ingredient choices, we were able to make over the most-beloved **Gooseberry Patch** slow-cooker main dish recipes and slash their calories to 400 or less. As a bonus, we've branched out beyond mains to include luscious desserts and snacks...most have less than 250 calories. Here's how we revamped the recipes:

- Used 2% reduced-fat milk instead of whole milk
- Substituted reduced-fat cheeses for regular cheeses or used full-fat cheeses in reduced amounts
- Used real butter in reduced amounts
- Trimmed fat from large cuts of beef
- Used skinless chicken breasts and chicken thighs
- Used lean ground beef and sausage
- Replaced thick-cut bacon with center-cut bacon
- Reduced meat, pork and poultry serving sizes to 6 ounces or less
- Reduced cooked grain and pasta portion sizes to ½ cup

With convenient and practically hands-free recipes for every meal of the day, you'll discover how easy it will be to stick to your healthy eating goals. We'll help you tackle serving ideas to keep your diet in check, so all you have to do is enjoy the results.

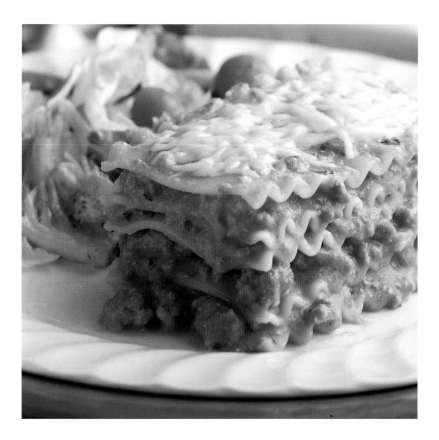

Inside you'll find:

Low-Cal Add-Ons provide calorie amounts for optional garnishes, side dishes and other accompaniments.

Skinny Secrets teach you the tricks and techniques to making lighter dishes without losing an ounce of lip-smacking taste.

Savvy Swaps give you ideas for handy, equal-calorie ingredient substitutions.

Nutrition Facts with every recipe provide a complete list of nutrients...including calories, total fat, saturated fat, cholesterol, sodium, carbohydrate, fiber and protein.

Whether you wish to get trim or simply maintain a balanced lifestyle, **Gooseberry Patch** *400-Calorie Slow-Cooker Recipes* takes the guesswork out of making calorie-controlled dishes your family will want to sink their teeth into, again and again.

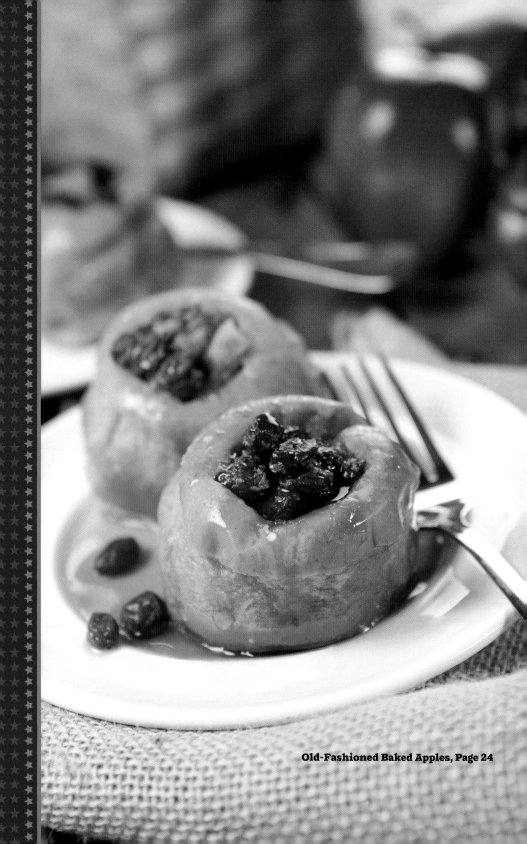

Old-Fashioned Baked Apples, Page 24

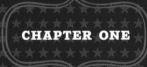

CHAPTER ONE

Breakfast & Brunch

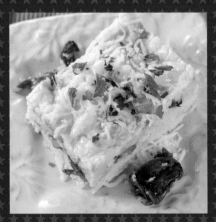

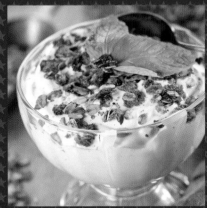

Mushroom & Cheese Strata, Page 10   Cinnamon-Cocoa Granola, Page 18

Jo Ann, Gooseberry Patch

Crustless Broccoli Quiche

This is a very versatile recipe...in springtime I like to use asparagus instead of broccoli. It's a great way to use up leftover shredded cheeses you may have in the fridge.

Makes 6 servings

6 eggs
2 T. all-purpose flour
1/2 t. salt
pepper to taste
1/8 t. nutmeg
1 c. half-and-half
1 c. 2% reduced-fat milk
3 c. cooked broccoli or other
  vegetable, chopped and well-
  drained
2 T. fresh basil, minced
1 c. shredded Gruyère cheese
1 c. shredded Parmesan cheese,
  divided

In a bowl, beat eggs with flour and seasonings; whisk in half-and-half and milk. Stir in broccoli, basil, Gruyère cheese and 1/2 cup Parmesan cheese. Spray a large slow cooker well with non-stick vegetable cooking spray. Pour egg mixture into slow cooker. Sprinkle remaining Parmesan cheese on top. Cover and cook on high setting for 1-1/2 hours, or until just set in the center. To serve, run a knife around the edge of quiche; cut into wedges.

Nutrition Per Serving: 294 calories, 19g total fat, 10g sat fat, 262mg cholesterol, 678mg sodium, 10g carbohydrate, 1g fiber, 21g protein

★ LOW-CAL ADD-ON ★ Round out your meal with a cup of mixed fresh blueberries and sliced fresh strawberries for only 70 calories per serving.

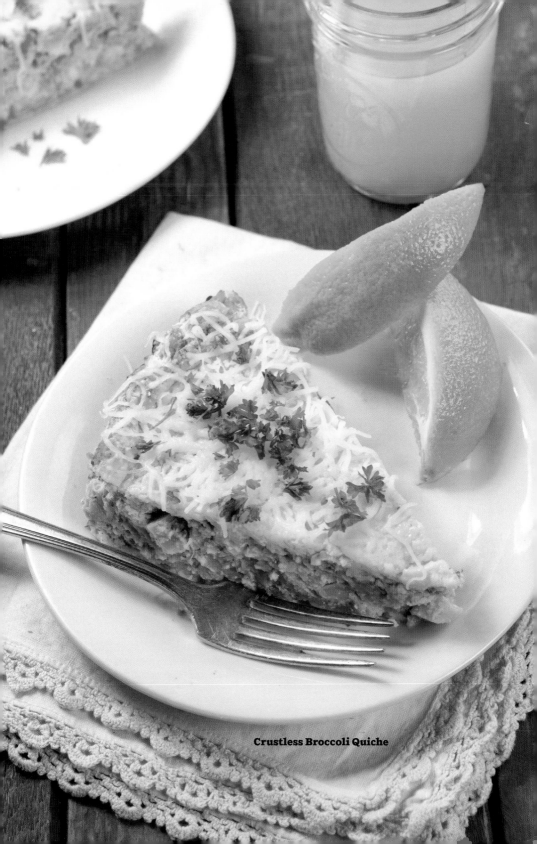

Crustless Broccoli Quiche

Connie Hilty, Pearland, TX

Breakfast Burritos

My teenage boys are always hungry, it seems! I love this recipe because it's so simple to fix and makes a lot. They love being able to grab a couple burritos, wrap them up and head for the school bus.

Makes 15 servings

20-oz. pkg. refrigerated diced
   potatoes, divided
8 slices center-cut bacon, crisply
   cooked, crumbled and divided
1/2 lb. lean ground turkey
   breakfast sausage, browned,
   drained and divided
2 c. shredded reduced-fat Cheddar
   cheese, divided
1/2 c. green pepper, diced
1/2 c. onion, diced
1 doz. eggs
1 c. 2% reduced-fat milk
3/4 t. salt
15 burrito-size flour tortillas
Garnish: salsa

Spray a large slow cooker well with non-stick vegetable spray. Layer half each of potatoes, bacon, sausage and cheese in slow cooker. Add all of green pepper and onion. Repeat layering, ending with cheese; set aside. In a large bowl, whisk together eggs, milk and salt; pour over layers in slow cooker. Cover and cook on low setting for 7 to 8 hours. To serve, spoon mixture into tortillas; garnish as desired and roll up.

Nutrition Per Serving: 309 calories, 13g total fat, 5g sat fat, 194mg cholesterol, 870mg sodium, 31g carbohydrate, 2g fiber, 17g protein

Rita Morgan, Pueblo, CO

Mexican Breakfast Casserole

I first tried this recipe when I was planning a church breakfast potluck... it was a hit! Now I serve it often.

Makes 8 servings

9 taco-size corn tortillas, divided
1 red pepper, diced and divided
3/4 c. green onions, sliced and divided
8-oz. pkg. shredded reduced-fat
   Mexican-blend cheese, divided
1 lb. lean ground turkey breakfast
   sausage, browned, drained
   and divided
8 eggs
1-1/2 c. 2% reduced-fat milk
1 T. canned diced green chiles, drained
1 to 2 T. fresh cilantro, chopped
Garnish: salsa

Spray a large slow cooker well with non-stick vegetable spray. Arrange 3 tortillas to cover the bottom of slow cooker, tearing to fit as needed; set aside. Reserve 2 tablespoons red pepper, 2 tablespoons green onions and 3/4 cup cheese; refrigerate. To slow cooker, add half of sausage and half each of remaining red pepper, green onions and cheese. Add 3 more tortillas, torn to fit; repeat layers. Top with remaining tortillas, tearing as needed to cover mixture. In a large bowl, whisk together eggs, milk and chiles; pour mixture over top. Cover and cook on low setting for 4 to 5 hours, or on high setting for 2 to 3 hours, until set in the center. Top with reserved cheese, pepper and onions; add cilantro. Serve with salsa.

Nutrition Per Serving: 357 calories, 18g total fat, 7g sat fat, 296mg cholesterol, 889mg sodium, 19g carbohydrate, 2g fiber, 30g protein

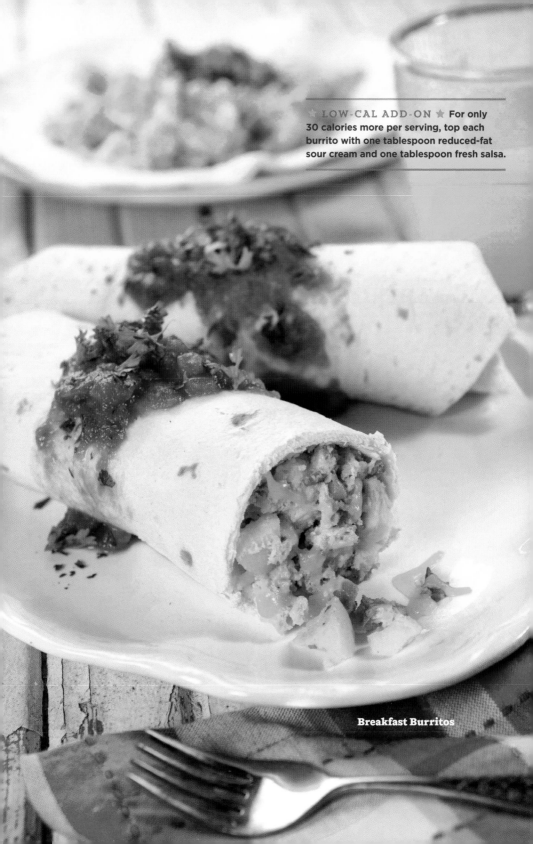

★ LOW-CAL ADD-ON ★ For only
30 calories more per serving, top each
burrito with one tablespoon reduced-fat
sour cream and one tablespoon fresh salsa.

Breakfast Burritos

Angela Murphy, Tempe, AZ

Mushroom & Cheese Strata

A brunch favorite! I keep a bag in the freezer for extra slices of bread, then when I have enough, I treat the family.

Makes 8 servings

1/2 lb. sliced mushrooms
1 T. olive oil
5 c. day-old Italian or white bread, cut into 1-inch cubes and divided
2 c. shredded Swiss cheese, divided
8 eggs
2-1/2 c. 2% reduced-fat milk
2 T. fresh thyme, snipped
1 T. Dijon mustard
1/4 t. salt
pepper to taste

In a skillet over medium heat, sauté mushrooms in oil for about 5 minutes, until mushrooms are softened and liquid is evaporated. Spray a slow cooker generously with non-stick vegetable spray. Spread 1/3 of bread in slow cooker; spoon half of mushrooms over bread and top with 1/3 of cheese. Repeat layering with half of remaining bread, remaining mushrooms and half of remaining cheese. Top with remaining bread; set aside. In a large bowl, beat together eggs, milk, thyme, mustard, salt and pepper; pour over bread. Gently press down bread to absorb egg mixture. Sprinkle remaining cheese on top. Cover and cook on low setting for 7 to 8 hours. Uncover; let stand for 15 minutes before serving.

Nutrition Per Serving: 270 calories, 15g total fat, 7g sat fat, 153mg cholesterol, 426mg sodium, 17g carbohydrate, 1g fiber, 17g protein

★ LOW-CAL ADD-ON ★ Sprinkle each serving with chopped fresh parsley for a boost in flavor and color without any extra calories.

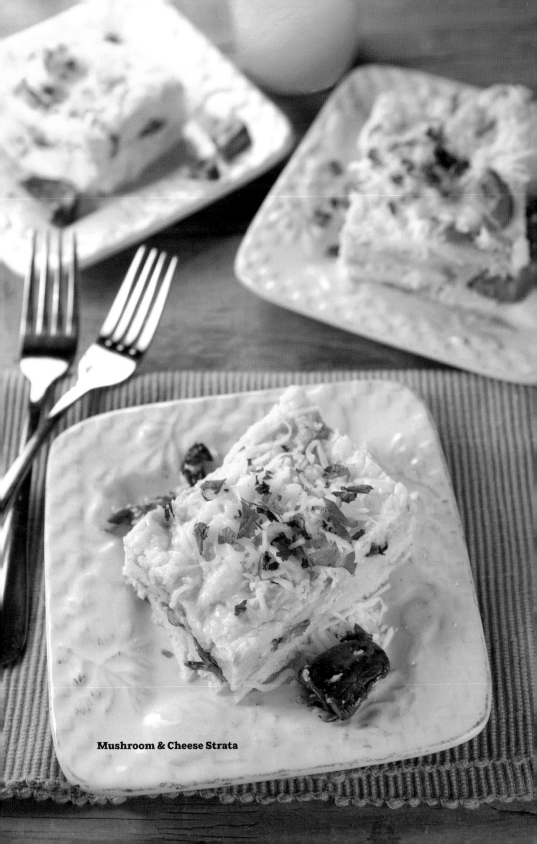

Mushroom & Cheese Strata

BREAKFAST & BRUNCH

Kelly Alderson, Erie, PA

Cheddar Cheese Strata

My favorite egg recipe for late-morning brunches. Sometimes we enjoy it as a breakfast-for-dinner too.

Makes 8 servings

3 c. 2% reduced-fat milk
14 1-oz. slices white bread, torn and divided
2 c. shredded reduced-fat sharp Cheddar cheese, divided
1/4 c. butter, diced and divided
6 eggs, beaten
2 T. Worcestershire sauce
1/2 t. salt
paprika to taste

Warm milk in a saucepan over low heat just until bubbles form; remove from heat. In a well-greased slow cooker, layer half each of bread, cheese and butter; set aside. In a bowl, whisk together warm milk and remaining ingredients except paprika. Pour into slow cooker; sprinkle with paprika. Cover and cook on low setting for 4 to 6 hours, until set.

Nutrition Per Serving: 361 calories, 19g total fat, 10g sat fat, 204mg cholesterol, 803mg sodium, 28g carbohydrate, 1g fiber, 20g protein

★ SAVVY SWAP ★ Use Swiss cheese instead of Cheddar for a milder flavor.

Patricia Wissler, Harrisburg, PA

Sausage & Egg Casserole

My children always loved having this casserole for breakfast on Sunday mornings. We like the mustard, but you may omit it if you prefer.

Makes 12 servings

1 T. butter, softened
14 1-1/2 oz. slices white bread
2 t. mustard
1 lb. lean ground turkey breakfast sausage, browned, drained and divided
2-1/2 c. shredded reduced-fat Cheddar or Monterey Jack cheese, divided
1 doz. eggs
2-1/4 c. 2% reduced-fat milk
1/2 t. salt
1 t. pepper, or to taste

Spread butter generously in a slow cooker; set aside. Spread bread slices with mustard on one side; cut bread into large squares. In slow cooker, layer 1/3 each of bread pieces, sausage and cheese. Repeat layering twice, ending with cheese on top. In a large bowl, beat together eggs, milk, salt and pepper; pour over cheese. Cover and cook on low setting for 8 to 9 hours, until set.

Nutrition Per Serving: 352 calories, 16g total fat, 6g sat fat, 271mg cholesterol, 905mg sodium, 26g carbohydrate, 1g fiber, 26g protein

Felice Jones, Boise, ID

Slow-Cooker Breakfast Casserole

This a perfect recipe for busy mornings. You wake up, the house smells so good and breakfast is ready as soon as you are.

Makes 10 servings

32-oz. pkg. frozen diced potatoes, divided
12 slices center-cut bacon, diced, crisply cooked and divided
1 onion, diced and divided
1 green pepper, diced and divided
1/2 c. shredded Monterey Jack cheese, divided
1 doz. eggs
1 c. 2% reduced-fat milk
1 t. salt
1 t. pepper

Layer 1/3 each of potatoes, bacon, onion, green pepper and cheese. Repeat layers 2 more times, ending with a layer of cheese; set aside. In a bowl, beat together eggs, milk, salt and pepper. Pour over mixture in slow cooker. Cover and cook on low setting for 8 to 9 hours.

Nutrition Per Serving: 239 calories, 10g total fat, 4g sat fat, 268mg cholesterol, 542mg sodium, 22g carbohydrate, 2g fiber, 15g protein

★ SKINNY SECRET ★ Center-cut bacon keeps the calories in check while still giving a smoky pop to each bite.

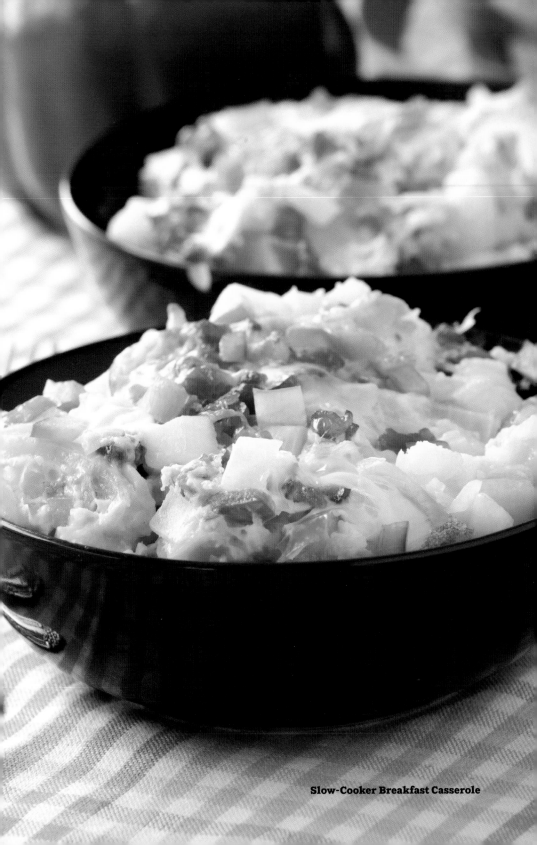

Slow-Cooker Breakfast Casserole

Rebecca McKeich,

Palm Beach Gardens, FL

Bacon-Hashbrown Breakfast Casserole

Every Christmas morning, our whole extended family descends upon our house to see what Santa has brought. It is our tradition to eat breakfast before we dive under the tree. After a couple years of making breakfast from scratch for a large group first thing in the morning, I came up with this. Prep it beforehand, toss it in the slow cooker before bed and you've got breakfast ready when you wake up. Just add coffee!

Makes 8 servings

26-oz. pkg. frozen shredded
   hashbrowns, thawed
12 slices center-cut bacon, crisply
   cooked and crumbled
2 c. shredded reduced-fat Cheddar
   cheese
1 doz. eggs
1 c. 2% reduced-fat milk
1 T. dry mustard
1/2 t. salt
pepper to taste

Spray a slow cooker generously with non-stick vegetable spray. Spread hashbrowns evenly in bottom of slow cooker. Top with bacon and cheese; set aside. In a large bowl, whisk together eggs, milk, mustard, salt and pepper. Pour over top and spread evenly. Cover and cook on low setting for 6 to 8 hours, until set.

Nutrition Per Serving: 352 calories, 19g total fat, 9g sat fat, 359mg cholesterol, 777mg sodium, 18g carbohydrate, 1g fiber, 27g protein

★ LOW-CAL ADD-ON ★ Combine 8 cups arugula, 2 cups sliced apples, 1/2 cup toasted walnut halves and 1/2 cup balsamic vinaigrette for a sweet, 90-calorie per serving companion to this hearty casserole.

Vickie, Gooseberry Patch

Overnight Blueberry French Toast

Sweetly satisfying! A perfect dish to make when you have overnight guests.

Makes 8 servings

1 c. brown sugar, packed
1-1/4 t. cinnamon
1/4 c. butter, melted
12 1-oz. slices white bread, divided
1-1/2 c. fresh or frozen blueberries
5 eggs
1-1/2 c. 2% reduced-fat milk
1 t. vanilla extract
1/2 t. salt
Garnish: whipped cream, additional
   blueberries

Combine brown sugar, cinnamon and melted butter in a bowl; mix well. Sprinkle 1/3 of mixture evenly in the bottom of a greased slow cooker. Cover with 6 bread slices. Sprinkle with another 1/3 of brown sugar mixture. Spread blueberries on top. Cover with remaining bread slices. Sprinkle with remaining brown sugar mixture and set aside. In a large bowl, whisk together eggs, milk, vanilla and salt; pour evenly over top. Press down gently on bread slices with a spoon. Cover and refrigerate overnight. In the morning, place crock into the slow cooker. Cover and cook on low setting 3 to 4 hours, until set and golden on top. Serve topped with a dollop of whipped cream and a few berries.

Nutrition Per Serving: 351 calories, 11g total fat, 6g sat fat, 153mg cholesterol, 472mg sodium, 54g carbohydrate, 2g fiber, 9g protein

★ SAVVY SWAP ★ Sliced fresh strawberries make a good sub for the blueberries.

Melody Taynor, Everette, WA

Cinnamon-Cocoa Granola

Try this healthy cereal with milk or sprinkled over nonfat Greek yogurt.

Makes 12 servings

4 c. long-cooking oats, uncooked
2/3 c. honey
1 c. bran cereal
1 c. wheat germ
1/2 c. sesame seeds
1/4 c. oil
2 T. baking cocoa
1 t. cinnamon

Combine all ingredients in a slow cooker. Cover and cook on low setting with lid slightly ajar for about 4 hours, stirring occasionally. Cool; store in an airtight container for one to 2 weeks.

Nutrition Per Serving: 271 calories, 10g total fat, 1g sat fat, 0mg cholesterol, 23mg sodium, 37g carbohydrate, 6g fiber, 8g protein

Tyson Ann Trecannelli,
Gettysburg, PA

Apple-Brown Sugar Oats

Even your picky eaters will love this one!

Makes 6 servings

2 c. 2% reduced-fat milk
1 c. long-cooking oats, uncooked
1 c. apple, peeled, cored and diced
1/2 c. raisins
1/4 c. brown sugar, packed
1 T. butter, melted
1/2 t. cinnamon
1/4 t. salt
Optional: 1/2 c. chopped walnuts
Garnish: 6 T. additional milk

Spray a slow cooker with non-stick vegetable spray. Add all ingredients except garnish; stir to mix well. Cover and cook on low setting overnight, about 8 hours. Spoon oatmeal into bowls; top with milk.

Nutrition Per Serving: 191 calories, 2g total fat, 3g sat fat, 12mg cholesterol, 59mg sodium, 38g carbohydrate, 2g fiber, 5g protein

★ LOW-CAL ADD-ON ★ Stir in chopped walnuts for some crunch and additional milk for more creaminess...these extras will only add 70 calories per serving.

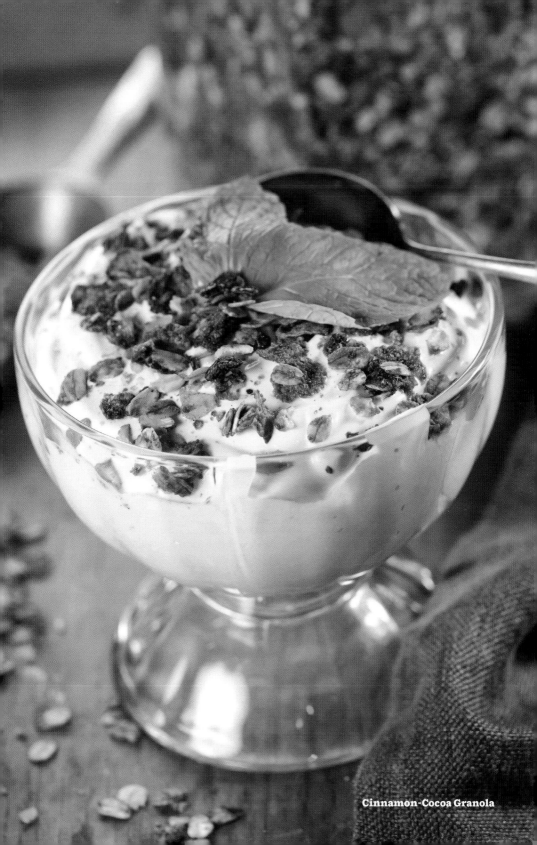

Cinnamon-Cocoa Granola

Joyceann Dreibelbis, Wooster, OH

Raisin-Nut Oatmeal

What's better than waking up to a ready-to-eat hot breakfast? The oats, fruit and spices in this homey meal bake together overnight.

Makes 6 servings

3-1/2 c. 2% reduced-fat milk
3/4 c. steel-cut oats, uncooked
1 Gala, Jonagold or Yellow Delicious
   apple, peeled, cored and diced
3/4 c. raisins
3 T. brown sugar, packed
4-1/2 t. butter, melted
3/4 t. cinnamon
1/4 c. chopped pecans

Spray a 3-quart slow cooker with non-stick vegetable spray. Add all ingredients except pecans; stir gently. Cover and cook on low setting for 7 to 8 hours, until liquid is absorbed. Spoon oatmeal into bowls; sprinkle with pecans.

Nutrition Per Serving: 300 calories, 10g total fat, 4g sat fat, 19mg cholesterol, 94mg sodium, 45g carbohydrate, 4g fiber, 8g protein

★ SAVVY SWAP ★ Substitute dried cranberries for the raisins if you like.

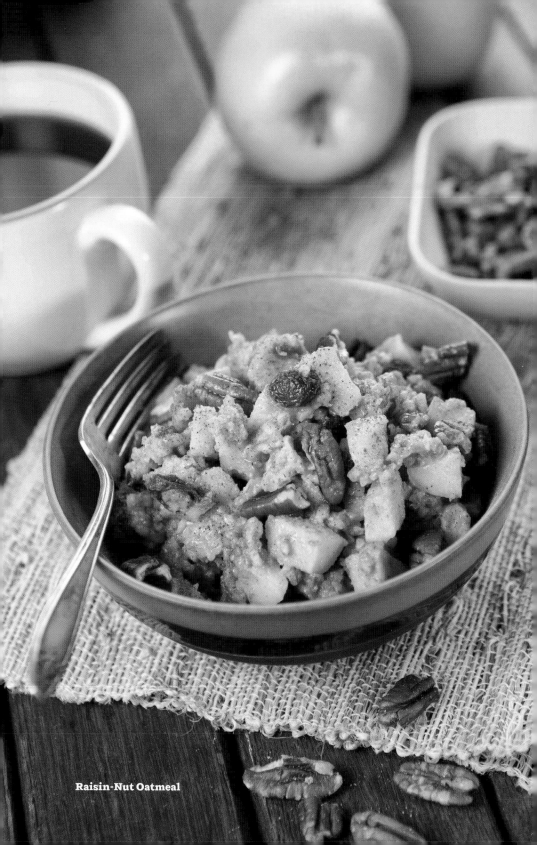

Raisin-Nut Oatmeal

Zoe Bennett, Columbia, SC

Cheesy Southern Grits

Dress up these southern-style grits with chopped green onion when serving a crowd. Cheddar cheese and milk makes them super creamy. Yummy!

Makes 8 servings

1-1/2 c. stone-ground or regular
   long-cooking grits, uncooked
6 c. water
1 c. 2% reduced-fat milk
2 T. butter, softened
1 t. salt
Optional: small amount of milk
1 c. shredded reduced-fat sharp
   Cheddar cheese

In a slow cooker, combine all ingredients except optional milk and cheese. Cover and cook on low setting for 6 to 8 hours, stirring occasionally. If mixture starts to dry out, stir in a little milk. About 15 to 30 minutes before serving time, stir in cheese; cover and finish cooking.

Nutrition Per Serving: 178 calories, 7g total fat, 4g sat fat, 20mg cholesterol, 443mg sodium, 22g carbohydrate, 2g fiber, 7g protein

★ SKINNY SECRET ★ Stirring the cheese into the grits during the last 15 to 30 minutes of cooking is the key to this dish's creamy texture.

Shelley Turner, Boise ID

Family-Favorite Potatoes

Packed with bacon and cheese, these potatoes are our favorite for weekend breakfasts. We love them at dinnertime too.

Makes 6 servings

3 lbs. russet potatoes, peeled, cubed
    and divided
1/4 c. onion, chopped and divided
1/2 t. salt
1/2 t. pepper
2 T. butter, diced and divided
6 slices center-cut bacon, crisply
    cooked, crumbled and divided
1 c. shredded Cheddar cheese,
    divided

Spray a large slow cooker with non-stick vegetable spray. Layer half each of potatoes and onion; sprinkle with salt and pepper. Add half each of remaining ingredients. Repeat layering, ending with cheese. Cover and cook on low setting for 8 to 10 hours, until potatoes are tender.

Nutrition Per Serving: 299 calories, 10g total fat, 6g sat fat, 26mg cholesterol, 497mg sodium, 39g carbohydrate, 3g fiber, 13g protein

Marsha Baker, Pioneer, OH

Old-Fashioned Baked Apples

I love these easy baked apples stuffed with cranberries or raisins... real comfort food. The recipe is so versatile...sweeten with sugar, sweetener or honey. I prefer Gala apples, but McIntosh, Rome or Empire would be delicious too. This recipe will bring raves!

Makes 6 servings

4 Gala apples
1/3 c. water
6 T. dark brown sugar, packed
4 T. sweetened dried cranberries or raisins
2 to 3 t. cinnamon, allspice or nutmeg, to taste
6 t. butter, sliced
Optional: honey or agave nectar to taste

Core each apple, leaving the base intact. Peel a one-inch strip from around the top of each apple. Arrange apples in a slow cooker. Add water; set aside. In a small bowl, combine sugar, cranberries or raisins and spice; stir until combined. Stuff each apple with brown sugar mixture, filling all the way to the top and pressing down to make room for more. Top each apple with a slice of butter. Drizzle apples with honey or agave nectar, if desired. Cover and cook on low setting for 3 to 4 hours, or on high setting for 2 to 3 hours, until apples are tender. Serve apples warm, drizzled with some of the syrup from the slow cooker.

Nutrition Per Serving: 165 calories, 4g total fat, 2g sat fat, 10mg cholesterol, 32mg sodium, 37g carbohydrate, 3g fiber, 0g protein

Donna Maltman, Toledo, OH

Country Sausage & Apples

A truly delicious slow-cooker recipe. There's just something about the combination of sausage and apples that tastes so good!.

Makes 8 servings

14-oz. pkg. smoked turkey sausage, sliced into 1-inch pieces
3 Granny Smith apples, cored and diced
1 c. brown sugar, packed
1/4 c. water

Place sausage in a slow cooker; top with apples. Sprinkle with brown sugar and drizzle water over all. Stir gently; cover and cook on high setting for 1-1/2 to 2 hours, until apples are tender.

Nutrition Per Serving: 247 calories, 10g total fat, 3g sat fat, 65mg cholesterol, 932mg sodium, 24g carbohydrate, 2g fiber, 15g protein

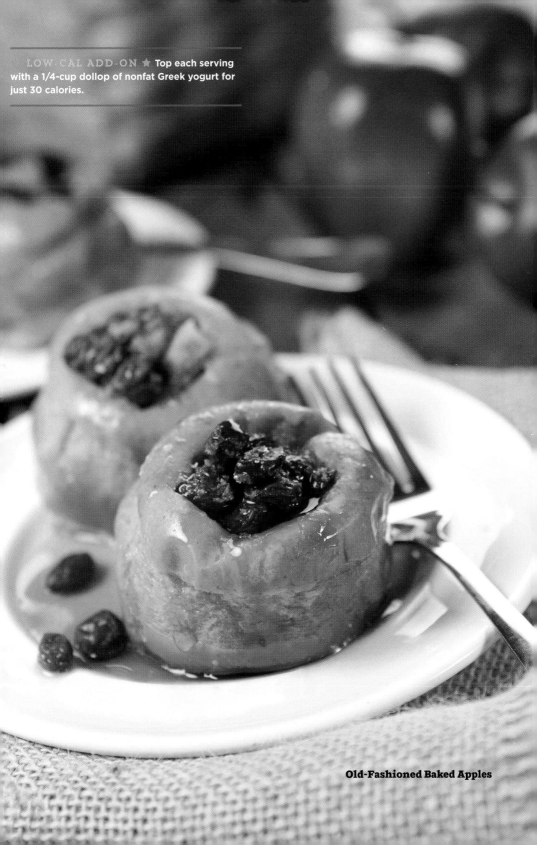

LOW-CAL ADD-ON ★ Top each serving with a 1/4-cup dollop of nonfat Greek yogurt for just 30 calories.

Old-Fashioned Baked Apples

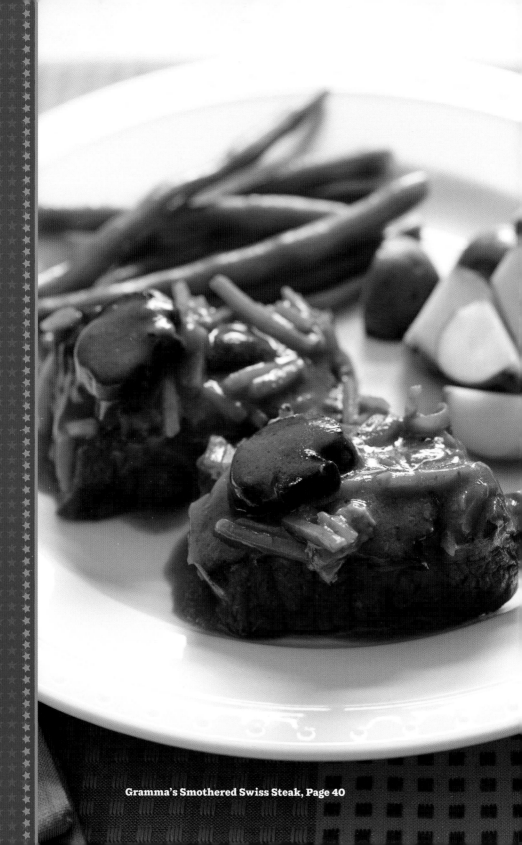

Gramma's Smothered Swiss Steak, Page 40

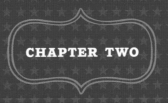

CHAPTER TWO

Beef

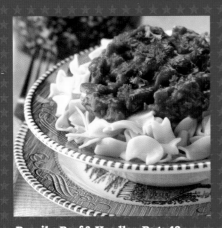

Paprika Beef & Noodles, Page 42

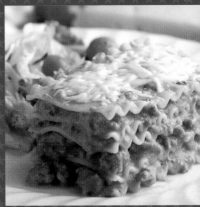

Best-Ever Lasagna, Page 48

Jessica Kraus, Delaware, OH

Braised Beef

Put this delicious recipe into your slow cooker in the morning and forget about it until dinnertime. Top each serving with chopped fresh basil for a bright burst of green color.

Makes 8 servings

2-lb. beef rump roast, fat trimmed
1 t. salt
1 t. pepper
3 T. olive oil
2 28-oz. cans whole tomatoes
1/2 c. beef broth
3 T. tomato paste
1 yellow onion, diced
3 cloves garlic, minced
1 t. dried basil
1 t. dried oregano
2 bay leaves
2 c. cooked polenta

Season roast with salt and pepper; set aside. Heat olive oil in a large deep skillet over medium heat. Add roast; brown on all sides. Remove roast to a slow cooker sprayed with non-stick vegetable spray. Top with undrained tomatoes and remaining ingredients except polenta. Spoon some of the mixture over roast. Cover and cook on low setting for 7 to 8 hours, until roast is very tender. Remove roast to a plate and shred with 2 forks. Discard bay leaves. Return to mixture in slow cooker; stir. Cover and cook on low setting for 15 additional minutes. To serve, ladle beef mixture over cooked polenta.

Nutrition Per Serving: 340 calories, 10g total fat, 3g sat fat, 67mg cholesterol, 678mg sodium, 35g carbohydrate, 5g fiber, 28g protein

---

★ LOW-CAL ADD-ON ★ **Spoon this saucy beef over 1/2 cup cooked polenta for an additional 100 calories per serving.**

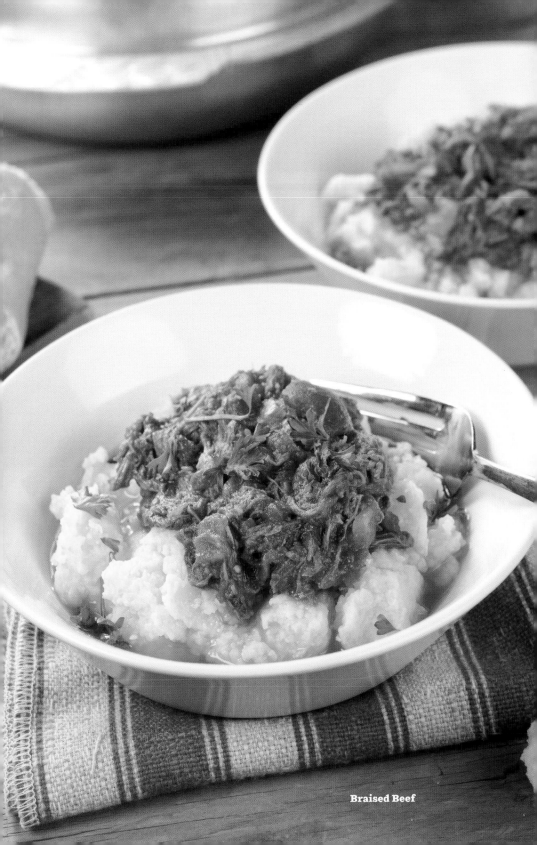

Braised Beef

Beverly Williams, San Antonio, TX

Pot Roast Dinner

This is one of my family's favorite dinners. The slow cooker makes it so easy for busy days.

Makes 6 servings

3-lb. boneless beef chuck roast,
   fat trimmed
1 t. garlic powder
3 c. beef broth, divided
2 russet potatoes, peeled and cubed
4 carrots, peeled and sliced
1 T. dried basil
1 t. dried oregano

Sprinkle roast evenly with garlic powder. Place in a slow cooker; add 2 cups broth. Cover and cook on high setting for 3-1/2 hours. Add potatoes, carrots, herbs and remaining broth to slow cooker. Cover and continue cooking on high setting for one additional hour, or until roast and vegetables are tender.

Nutrition Per Serving: 351 calories, 10g total fat, 4g sat fat, 132mg cholesterol, 552mg sodium, 18g carbohydrate, 3g fiber, 47g protein

Rita Morgan, Pueblo, CO

Farmhouse Pot Roast

After all day in the slow cooker, this roast is falling-apart tender and makes its own gravy.

Makes 6 servings

3-lb. boneless beef chuck roast,
   fat trimmed
4-oz. can sliced mushrooms, drained
6 redskin potatoes, cubed
1/2 lb. baby carrots
3 stalks celery, chopped
14-1/2 oz. can beef broth
2 c. water
26-oz. can cream of mushroom soup

Place roast in a large slow cooker; top with vegetables. In a bowl, blend together broth, water and soup; pour over roast. Cover and cook on low setting for 8 hours, or until roast is very tender.

Nutrition Per Serving: 369 calories, 8g total fat, 3g sat fat, 103mg cholesterol, 572mg sodium, 35g carbohydrate, 5g fiber, 39g protein

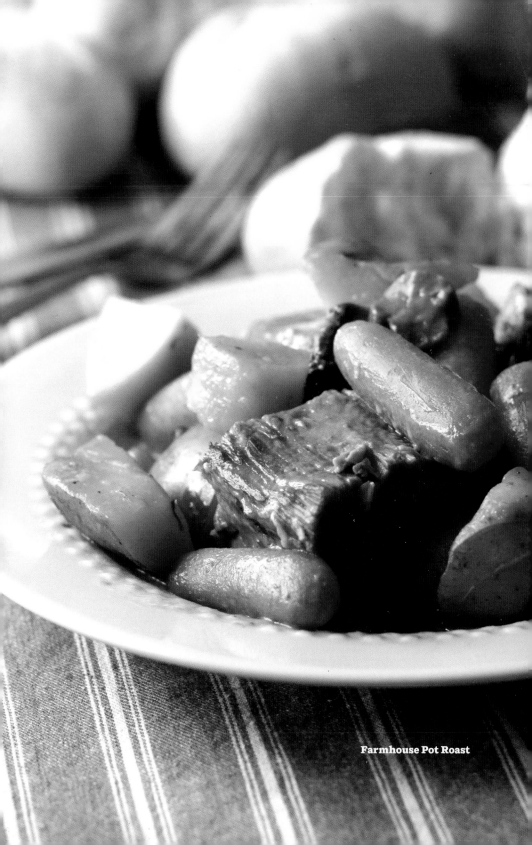

Farmhouse Pot Roast

Jill Burton, Gooseberry Patch

Tomasso's Italian Beef

My brother-in-law is from Italy and is a fabulous cook! He served this at a family reunion, where it was an instant hit.

Makes 6 servings

10-3/4 oz. can tomato soup
10-1/2 oz. can beef broth
1/2 c. dry red wine or water
2 lbs. stew beef cubes
14-1/2 oz. can diced Italian-style tomatoes
3 carrots, peeled and cut into 1-inch pieces
1 t. Italian seasoning
1/2 t. garlic powder
2 16-oz. cans cannellini beans, drained and rinsed

Combine all ingredients except beans in a slow cooker. Cover and cook on low setting for 6 to 8 hours, or on high setting for 3 to 5 hours. Stir in beans. Turn setting to high; cover and cook for an additional 10 minutes, or until beans are warmed through.

Nutrition Per Serving: 333 calories, 7g total fat, 3g sat fat, 98mg cholesterol, 830mg sodium, 28g carbohydrate, 6g fiber, 40g protein

★ LOW-CAL ADD-ON ★ **Pair each serving with a warm, one-ounce slice of bread from a baguette for 70 more calories.**

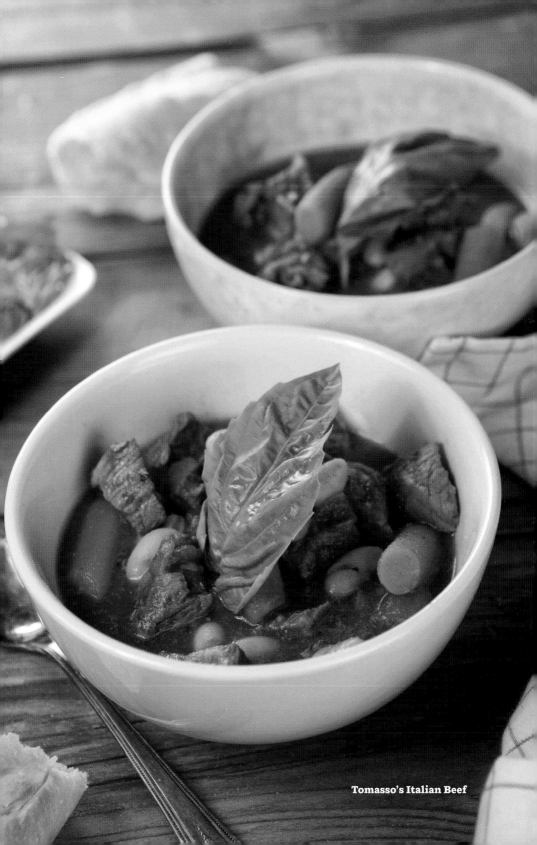

Tomasso's Italian Beef

Erin Gumm, Omaha, NE

Slow-Cooker Fajitas

These are always a favorite for casual dinner parties or when the whole family gets together...and the slow cooker does all the work!

Makes 8 servings

1-1/2 lbs. lean beef round steak
8-oz. can diced tomatoes, drained
1 onion, sliced
1 green pepper, cut into strips
1 red pepper, cut into strips
1 jalapeño pepper, chopped
1 t. fresh cilantro, chopped
2 cloves garlic, minced
1 t. chili powder
1 t. ground cumin
1 t. ground coriander
1/4 t. salt
12 6-inch whole-wheat flour
   tortillas
Garnish: reduced-fat sour cream,
   guacamole, salsa, reduced-fat
   shredded cheese, shredded lettuce

Place steak in a slow cooker. Combine vegetables and seasonings; spoon over steak. Cover and cook on low setting for 8 to 10 hours, or on high setting for 4 to 5 hours. Shred steak; serve with a slotted spoon on tortillas and garnish with favorite toppings.

Nutrition Per Serving: 375 calories, 13g total fat, 6g sat fat, 78mg cholesterol, 496mg sodium, 33g carbohydrate, 6g fiber, 32g protein

★ LOW-CAL ADD-ON ★ Top fajitas with one teaspoon each of sour cream, cheese and guacamole for only 25 more calories per serving.

Panda Spurgin, Berryville, AK

Slow-Cooker Enchiladas

This came from a friend that I worked with. We were always exchanging recipes to have on hand for busy days.

Makes 6 servings

1 lb. lean ground beef
1 c. onion, chopped
1/2 c. green pepper, chopped
15-1/2 oz. can black beans, drained and rinsed
10-oz. can diced tomatoes with green chiles
1/3 c. water
1 t. chili powder
1/2 t. ground cumin
1/2 t. salt
1/4 t. pepper
1-1/2 c. shredded Monterey Jack cheese, divided
6 6-inch whole-wheat flour tortillas, divided
Garnish: salsa, reduced-fat sour cream

In a skillet over medium heat, brown beef, onion and pepper; drain. Stir in remaining ingredients except cheese, tortillas and garnish; bring to a simmer. Cook, stirring occasionally, until heated through, about 5 minutes. In a slow cooker, alternate layers of beef mixture, tortillas and cheese, ending with cheese. Cover and cook on low setting for 5 to 7 hours. Garnish servings as desired.

Nutrition Per Serving: 354 calories, 16g total fat, 9g sat fat, 73mg cholesterol, 880mg sodium, 24g carbohydrate, 5g fiber, 29g protein

---

★ SAVVY SWAP ★ Use lean ground turkey instead of ground beef.

Jenessa Yauch, Munhall, PA

Ropa Vieja

This is an old Cuban recipe which literally translates to "old clothes." It is very flavorful.

Makes 8 servings

1 T. olive oil
2-lb. beef flank steak or London broil
8-oz. can tomato sauce
6-oz. can tomato paste
1 c. beef broth
1/2 c. yellow onion, diced
1 green pepper, sliced into strips
1 T. vinegar
2 cloves garlic, minced
1 t. ground cumin
1 t. dried cilantro
4 c. cooked brown rice

Heat oil in a skillet over medium heat; brown beef on both sides. Drain; transfer to a slow cooker. Add remaining ingredients except rice; stir. Cover and cook on low setting for 8 hours, or on high setting for 4 hours, until beef is tender. Shred beef in slow cooker; stir well and serve over cooked rice.

Nutrition Per Serving: 335 calories, 4g total fat, 3g sat fat, 70mg cholesterol, 381mg sodium, 46g carbohydrate, 4g fiber, 29g protein

★ LOW-CAL ADD-ON ★ Top each portion with 2 tablespoons sliced pimento-stuffed olives for only 15 calories more per serving.

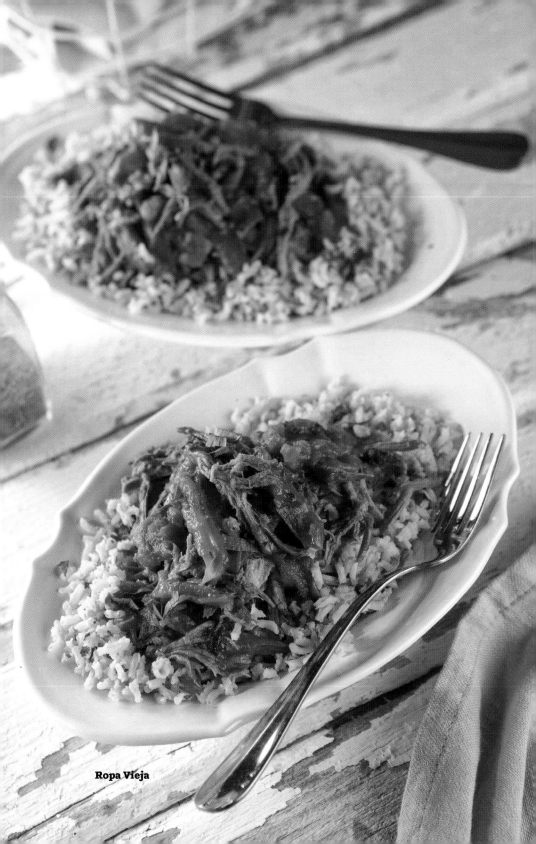

Ropa Vieja

Lee Beedle, Martinsburg, WV

Orange & Ginger Beef Short Ribs

Cooking short ribs in the slow cooker with a mixture of soy sauce and brown sugar makes the beef unbelievably tender and tasty.

Makes 8 servings.

1/3 c. reduced-sodium soy sauce
3 T. brown sugar, packed
3 T. white vinegar
2 cloves garlic, minced
1/2 t. chili powder
1 T. fresh ginger, peeled and minced
3 lbs. boneless lean beef short ribs
1/4 c. orange marmalade
4 c. cooked brown rice

In a large plastic zipping bag, combine all ingredients except ribs, marmalade and rice. Add ribs to bag; turn to coat. Refrigerate at least 2 hours to overnight. Drain ribs, reserving marinade. Place ribs in a slow cooker. Add marmalade to reserved marinade; mix well and pour over ribs. Cover and cook on low setting for 6 to 8 hours. Serve over brown rice.

Nutrition Per Serving: 395 calories, 14g total fat, 6g sat fat, 69mg cholesterol, 438mg sodium, 41g carbohydrate, 2g fiber, 26g protein

Debi Finnen, Berlin Heights, OH

Slow-Cooker Pepper Steak

This is a good recipe to make when onions and peppers are plentiful in your backyard garden.

Makes 8 servings

2 lbs. beef sirloin, cut into bite-size
   strips
garlic powder to taste
3 T. oil
1 cube beef bouillon
1/4 c. boiling water
1 T. cornstarch
1/2 c. onion, chopped
2 green peppers, thinly sliced
14-oz. can stewed tomatoes
3 T. reduced-sodium soy sauce
1 t. sugar
1 t. salt
4 c. cooked brown rice

Sprinkle beef with garlic powder. In a large skillet over medium heat, brown beef in oil. Transfer to a slow cooker. Mix together bouillon cube and water until dissolved; stir in cornstarch until dissolved. Pour over beef. Stir in remaining ingredients except rice. Cover and cook on low setting for 6 to 8 hours, or on high setting for 3 to 4 hours. Serve over rice.

Nutrition Per Serving: 357 calories, 11g total fat, 3g sat fat, 68mg cholesterol, 824mg sodium, 36g carbohydrate, 3g fiber, 29g protein

★ SAVVY SWAP ★ **Sub in broccoli flowerets and carrots for the peppers.**

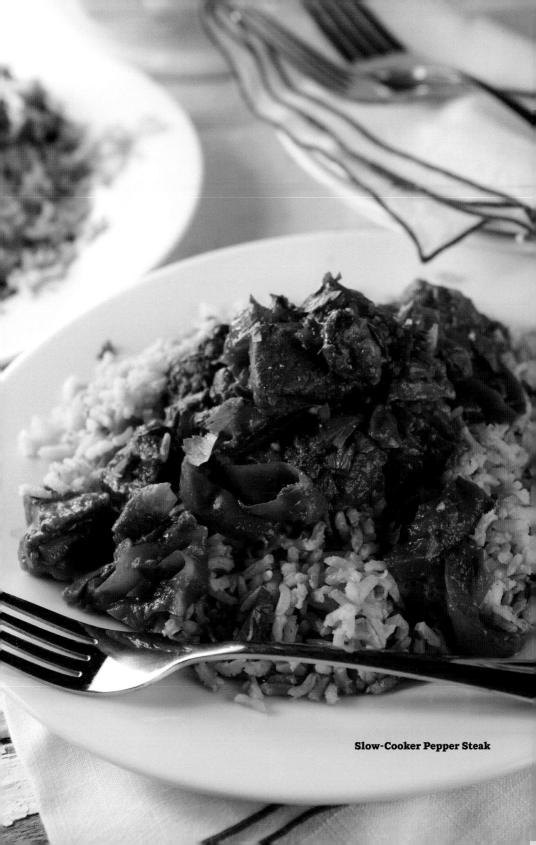

Slow-Cooker Pepper Steak

Jennifer Martineau, Delaware, OH

Gramma's Smothered Swiss Steak

So tender...yummy with mashed potatoes.

Makes 6 servings

1-1/2 lbs. beef round steak, cut into
    6 pieces
1 T. oil
1 small onion, halved and sliced
1 carrot, peeled and shredded
1 c. sliced mushrooms
10-3/4 oz. can low-sodium cream of
    mushroom soup
8-oz. can no-salt tomato sauce

Brown beef in oil in a skillet over medium heat; drain and set aside. Arrange vegetables in a slow cooker; place beef on top. Mix together soup and tomato sauce; pour over beef and vegetables. Cover and cook on low setting for 6 hours, or until beef is tender.

Nutrition Per Serving: 381 calories, 20g total fat, 8g sat fat, 111mg cholesterol, 237mg sodium, 14g carbohydrate, 1 fiber, 36g protein

★ LOW-CAL ADD-ON ★ **Spoon one cup steamed green beans onto your plate for only 60 extra calories.**

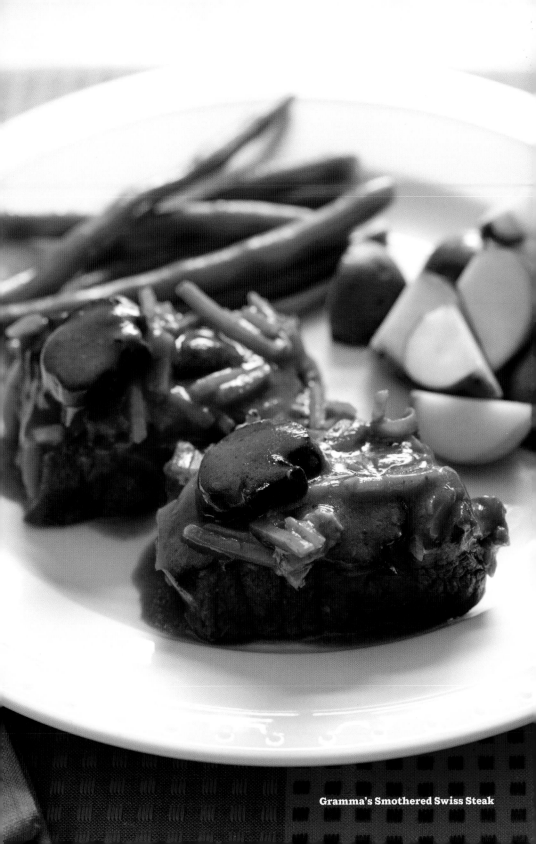

Gramma's Smothered Swiss Steak

Lisann Miller, Canton, MS

Irish Corned Beef Dinner

I make this for my family every year for St. Patrick's Day. Be sure to cut the vegetables all the same size so they'll cook evenly.

Makes 10 servings

3-lb. corned beef brisket
4 potatoes, quartered
3/4 lb. carrots, peeled, halved and cut into sticks
1 head cabbage, cut into wedges
2 onions, quartered
12-oz. can regular beer or non-alcoholic beer
1 bay leaf
2 to 3 c. water

Place corned beef brisket in a slow cooker. Arrange vegetables around brisket; add beer, bay leaf and enough water to cover. Cover and cook on low setting for 7 to 8 hours. Discard bay leaf. To serve, arrange vegetables on a large serving platter. Slice brisket and arrange over vegetables.

Nutrition Per Serving: 389 calories, 21g total fat, 7g sat fat, 74mg cholesterol, 1712mg sodium, 28g carbohydrate, 5g fiber, 24g protein

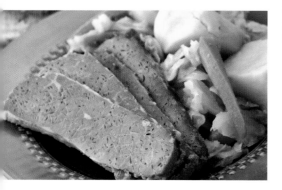

Teresa Pearman, Marshall NC

Paprika Beef & Noodles

This recipe is as good tasting as it is easy! We enjoy the fork-tender beef served over cooked egg noodles.

Makes 8 servings

1-3/4 c. water, divided
2 lbs. stew beef cubes
1 c. onion, sliced
1 clove garlic, diced
3/4 c. catsup
2 T. Worcestershire sauce
1 T. brown sugar, packed
2 t. salt
2 t. paprika
1/8 t. dry mustard
1/8 t. cayenne pepper
2 T. all-purpose flour
4 c. cooked egg noodles

In a slow cooker, combine 1-1/2 cups water and remaining ingredients except flour and noodles; mix well. Cover and cook on low setting for 6 to 8 hours. In a cup, stir together remaining water and flour. Drizzle into beef mixture; stir. Cook, uncovered, until thickened. Serve beef mixture over noodles.

Nutrition Per Serving: 290 calories, 6g total fat, 3g sat fat, 110mg cholesterol, 1020mg sodium, 30g carbohydrate, 1g fiber, 29g protein

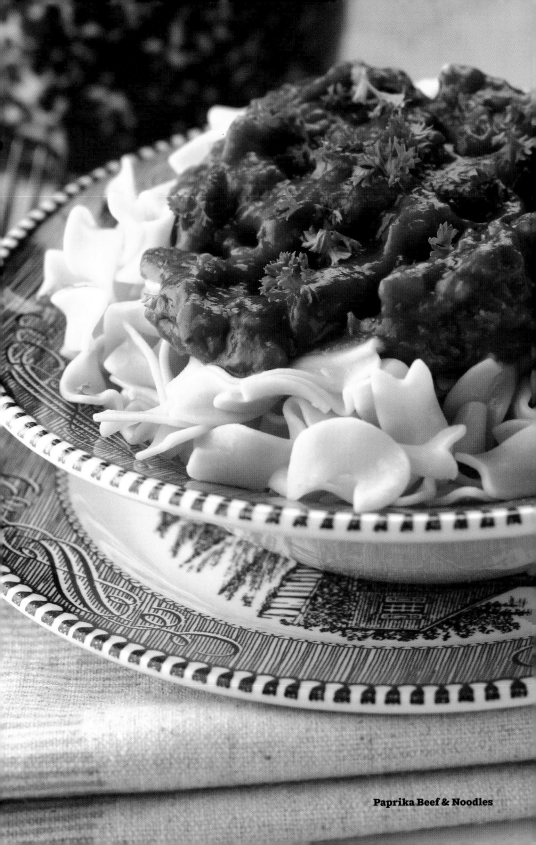

Paprika Beef & Noodles

Pamela Lome, Buffalo Grove, IL

Easy Beef Goulash

On cold days, this dish is wonderful to make in the morning and come home to find it waiting for you!

Makes 6 servings

1/2 c. all-purpose flour
1 T. paprika
1 t. salt
1 t. pepper
1-1/2 lbs. beef chuck steak, fat trimmed and cut into 1-inch cubes
1 T. olive oil
6-oz. can tomato paste
1/2 t. dried oregano
1/2 t. dried basil
1 small red onion, chopped

Combine flour, paprika, salt and pepper in a small bowl. Dredge beef cubes in mixture. Brown beef in hot oil in a skillet over medium heat. Place beef in a slow cooker; top with tomato paste, herbs and onion. Add just enough water to cover beef; stir to blend. Cover and cook on low setting for 5 to 6 hours.

Nutrition Per Serving: 387 calories, 23g total fat, 8g sat fat, 74mg cholesterol, 563mg sodium, 21g carbohydrate, 3g fiber, 24g protein protein

Vickie, Gooseberry Patch

Spaghetti Pie

An old favorite! Sometimes I layer sliced mushrooms and black olives with the other ingredients.

Makes 8 servings

8-oz. pkg. spaghetti, uncooked and broken up
1 lb. lean ground beef
32-oz. jar pasta sauce
2 eggs, beaten
1/3 c. grated Parmesan cheese
3 c. 2% reduced-fat cottage cheese, divided
1 c. shredded reduced-fat Italian-blend cheese, divided

Cook spaghetti according to package directions, just until tender; drain and return to pan. Meanwhile, brown beef in a skillet over medium heat; drain. Add sauce to beef; simmer over low heat for several minutes. To spaghetti in pan, add eggs and Parmesan cheese; stir gently to mix. Spoon 1/2 cup sauce mixture into a slow cooker. Layer with half each of spaghetti mixture, cottage cheese, remaining sauce mixture and shredded cheese. Repeat layering. Cover and cook on low setting for 8 to 6 hours.

Nutrition Per Serving: 343 calories, 10g total fat, 4g sat fat, 92mg cholesterol, 746mg sodium, 36g carbohydrate, 3g fiber, 27g protein

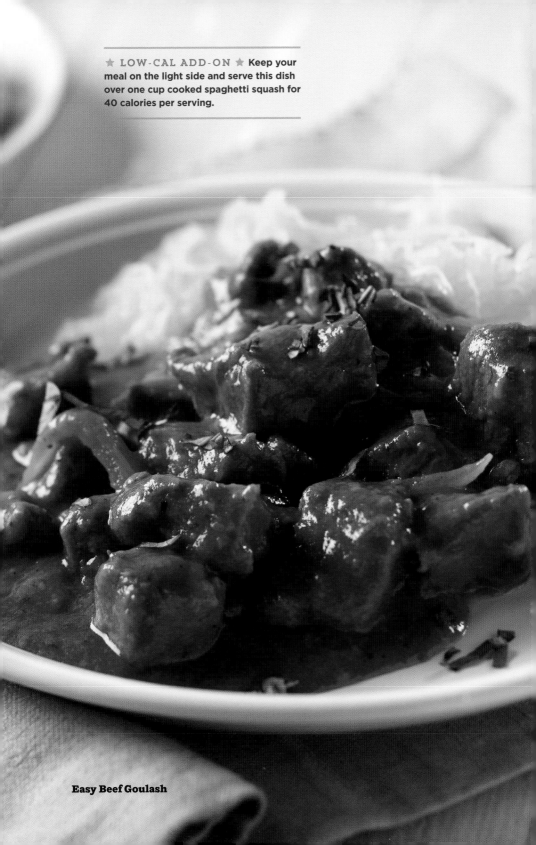

★ LOW-CAL ADD-ON ★ Keep your meal on the light side and serve this dish over one cup cooked spaghetti squash for 40 calories per serving.

Easy Beef Goulash

Kristi Magowan, Greenwich, NY

Bowtie Lasagna Casserole

This is always my go-to supper for when our whole family eats together.

Makes 10 servings

1 lb. lean ground beef
1 T. olive oil
1 onion, chopped
1 t. garlic, chopped
28-oz. can crushed tomatoes
8-oz. can tomato sauce
1 T. brown sugar, packed
1 T. dried oregano
1 t. salt
1 t. pepper
8-oz. pkg. bowtie pasta, uncooked
15-oz. container part-skim ricotta
   cheese
1 c. shredded part-skim mozzarella
   cheese
Garnish: grated Parmesan cheese

In a skillet over medium heat, cook beef until no longer pink. Drain; add to a slow cooker. Add olive oil and onion to skillet; cook until translucent, 5 to 7 minutes. Add garlic; cook for one minute. Spoon onion mixture over beef; stir in undrained tomatoes, tomato sauce, brown sugar, oregano, salt and pepper. Cover and cook at low setting for 6 to 7 hours. About 30 minutes before serving, cook pasta according to package directions; drain. Add cooked pasta and ricotta cheese to sauce in slow cooker; stir to combine. Top with mozzarella cheese. Turn slow cooker to high setting. Cover and cook for an additional 30 minutes, or until heated through and cheese is melted. Serve garnished with Parmesan cheese.

Nutrition Per Serving: 301 calories, 11g total fat, 5g sat fat, 50mg cholesterol, 635mg sodium, 29g carbohydrate, 3g fiber, 22g protein

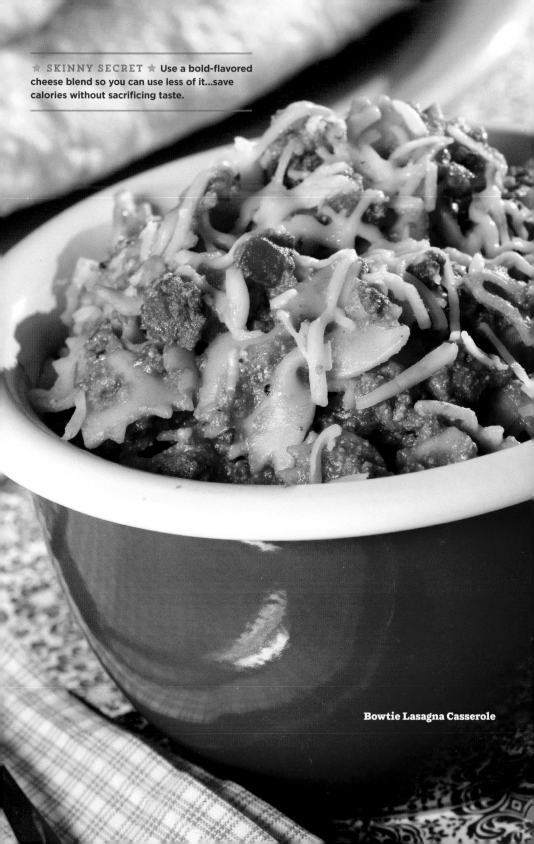

Bowtie Lasagna Casserole

Cherylann Smith, Efland, NC

Best-Ever Lasagna

This is a quick & easy recipe for homestyle lasagna...just add a tossed salad.

Makes 10 servings

1 lb. lean ground beef, browned and
    drained
1 t. Italian seasoning
8 lasagna noodles, uncooked and
    broken into thirds
28-oz. jar spaghetti sauce
1/3 c. water
4-oz. can sliced mushrooms, drained
15-oz. container part-skim ricotta
    cheese
8-oz. pkg. shredded part-skim
    mozzarella cheese
Garnish: shredded Parmesan cheese

Combine beef and Italian seasoning. Arrange half of the lasagna noodles in a slow cooker sprayed with non-stick vegetable spray. Spread half of beef mixture over noodles. Top with half each of remaining ingredients except Parmesan cheese. Repeat layering process. Cover and cook on low setting for 5 hours. Garnish with Parmesan cheese.

Nutrition Per Serving: 318 calories, 13g total fat, 6g sat fat, 60mg cholesterol, 593mg sodium, 26g carbohydrate, 2g fiber, 24g protein

★ LOW-CAL ADD-ON ★ Sprinkle each serving with one tablespoon shredded Parmesan cheese for just 25 more calories.

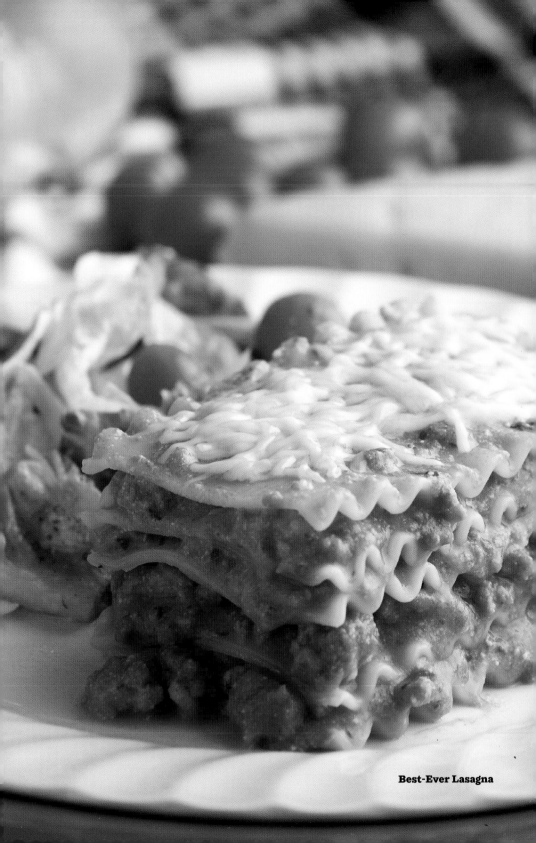

Best-Ever Lasagna

BEEF

JoAnn, Gooseberry Patch

Burgundy Meatloaf

So good...this is a main dish you can count on!

Makes 8 servings

2 lbs. lean ground beef
2 eggs
1 c. soft bread crumbs
1 onion, chopped
1/2 c. Burgundy wine or beef broth
1/2 c. fresh parsley, chopped
1 T. fresh basil, chopped
1-1/2 t. salt
1/4 t. pepper
5 slices center-cut bacon
1 bay leaf
8-oz. can tomato sauce

In a large bowl, combine beef, eggs, crumbs, onion, wine or broth and seasonings; mix well and set aside. Criss-cross 3 bacon slices on a 12-inch square of aluminum foil. Form beef mixture into a 6-inch round loaf on top of bacon. Cut remaining bacon slices in half; arrange on top of meatloaf. Place bay leaf on top. Lift meatloaf by aluminum foil into a slow cooker; cover and cook on high setting for one hour. Reduce to low setting; cover and and continue cooking for an additional 4 hours. Remove meatloaf from slow cooker by lifting foil. Place on a serving platter, discarding foil., bacon and bay leaf. Warm tomato sauce and spoon over sliced meatloaf.

Nutrition Per Serving: 273 calories, 14g total fat, 5g sat fat, 130mg cholesterol, 769mg sodium, 9g carbohydrate, 1g fiber, 28g protein

★ LOW-CAL ADD-ON ★ Serve with 1/2 cup each of roasted Brussels sprouts and red potatoes for only 100 calories per serving. You can bake them 20 minutes before the meatloaf finishes cooking.

Ida Mannion, North Chelmsford, MA

Stuffed Cabbage Rolls

This is a recipe my mom used to make for my dad. It was one of his favorite meals. They had eight children and this went a long way at mealtime. The vegetable juice is my own addition.

Makes 12 servings

1 head cabbage, cored
3/4-c. instant rice, uncooked
1 egg, lightly beaten
1/2 c. onion, diced
salt to taste
1-1/2 lbs. lean ground beef
46-oz. can cocktail vegetable juice

Add cabbage to a large pot of boiling water. Cook just until cabbage leaves fall off head. Drain well; set aside 12 large leaves for rolls. In a large bowl, combine uncooked rice, egg, onion and salt. Crumble uncooked beef over mixture and mix well. Place 1/3 cup beef mixture on each cabbage leaf; overlap ends of leaf and fold in sides. Roll up completely to enclose filling; secure with wooden toothpicks, if desired. Place cabbage rolls in a slow cooker. Pour vegetable juice over rolls. Cover and cook on low setting for 6 to 7 hours.

Nutrition Per Serving: 340 calories, 9g total fat, 4g sat fat, 107mg cholesterol, 508mg sodium, 35g carbohydrate, 7g fiber, 30g protein

Beth Kramer, Port Saint Lucie, FL

Fix & Forget Stuffed Peppers

Use red or yellow peppers for bright color and a milder taste.

Makes 6 servings

1 lb. lean ground beef
1 c. long-cooking rice, uncooked
1 onion, chopped
1 carrot, peeled and shredded
1 t. beef bouillon granules
1/2 t. salt
1/2 t. pepper
6 green peppers, tops removed
10-3/4 oz. can tomato soup
1-1/4 c. water

In a large bowl, combine beef, rice, onion, carrot, bouillon, salt and pepper. Stuff each green pepper about 2/3 full. Arrange peppers side-by-side in a slow cooker. Combine soup and water; pour over peppers. Cover and cook on low setting for 6 to 8 hours.

Nutrition Per Serving: 239 calories, 6g total fat, 2g sat fat, 49mg cholesterol, 551mg sodium, 27g carbohydrate, 3g fiber, 19g protein

★ SAVVY SWAP ★ You can use 1-1/4 cups beef broth instead of the water...just be sure to omit the bouillon in the beef mixture.

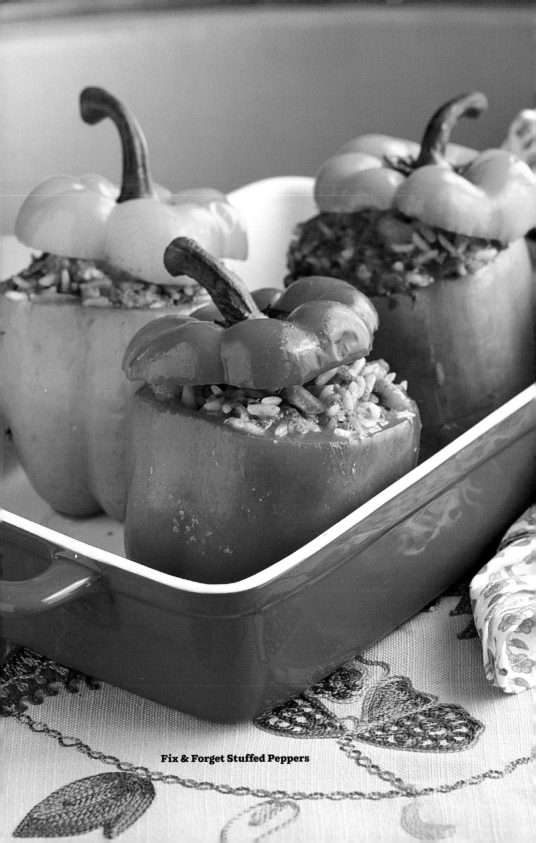

Fix & Forget Stuffed Peppers

Claire Bertram, Lexington KY

Beefy Mushroom Casserole

This is a dinner I can count on when time is short. I serve it with a simple side of steamed veggies to complete the meal.

Makes 6 servings

1-1/2 lbs. beef round steak, cubed
3/4 c. quick-cooking barley, uncooked
10-3/4 oz. can golden mushroom soup
2/3 c. water
3/4 lb. sliced mushrooms
Garnish: reduced-fat shredded
   cheese, diced green onions

Combine all ingredients except garnish in a slow cooker; mix well. Cover and cook on low setting for 7 to 8 hours. Garnish as desired.

Nutrition Per Serving: 260 calories, 7g total fat, 2g sat fat, 69mg cholesterol, 424mg sodium, 19g carbohydrate, 3g fiber, 30g protein

Sharon Crider, Lebanon, MO

Spanish Rice

Baked tortilla scoops are tasty to serve along this one-dish supper.

Makes 8 servings

2 lbs. lean ground beef, browned and
   drained
28-oz. can crushed tomatoes
8-oz. can tomato sauce
2 green peppers, chopped
2 onions, chopped
1 c. water
2-1/2 t. chili powder
2 t. Worcestershire sauce
1 t. salt
1 c. long-cooking rice, uncooked

Combine all ingredients in a slow cooker; mix well. Cover and cook on low setting for 6 to 8 hours, or on high setting for 3-1/2 hours.

Nutrition Per Serving: 319 calories, 8g total fat, 3g sat fat, 71mg cholesterol, 710mg sodium, 34g carbohydrate, 4g fiber, 28g protein

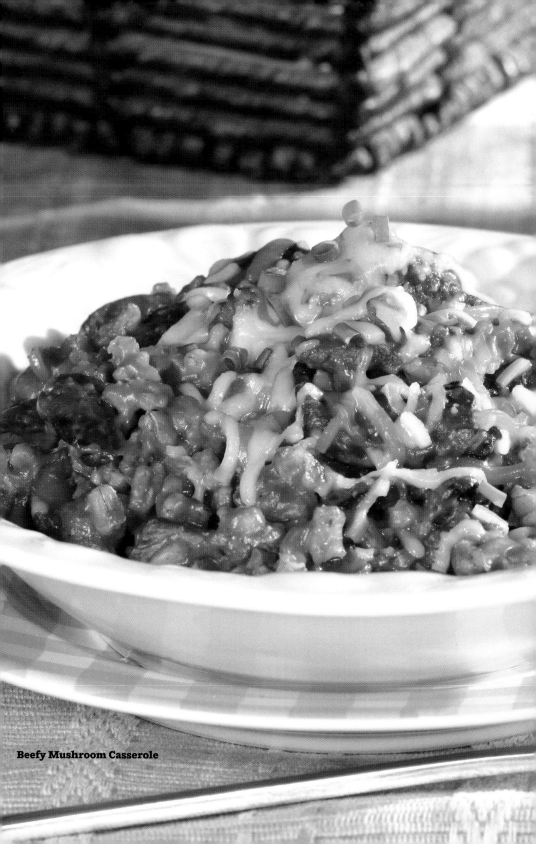

Beefy Mushroom Casserole

Carolyn Deckard, Bedford IN

Tamale Casserole

Another easy meal you can put together and let cook while you work or play. I always serve a lettuce salad with it.

Makes 6 servings

1 lb. lean ground beef
1 egg, beaten
1-1/2 c. 2% reduced-fat milk
3/4 c. cornmeal
14-1/2 oz. can diced tomatoes
15-1/4 oz. can corn, drained
2-1/2 oz. can sliced black olives, drained
1-oz. pkg. chili seasoning mix
1/2 t. seasoned salt
1 c. shredded reduced-fat Cheddar cheese

In a skillet over medium heat, cook beef until no longer pink; drain. Meanwhile, in a bowl, combine egg, milk and cornmeal. Stir until smooth; add tomatoes with juice, corn, olives, seasoning mix and seasoned salt. Add beef; stir well and spoon into a slow cooker sprayed with non-stick vegetable spray. Cover and cook on high setting for 3 hours and 45 minutes. Sprinkle with cheese. Cover and cook 15 minutes longer, or until cheese is melted.

Nutrition Per Serving: 343 calories, 12g total fat, 6g sat fat, 99mg cholesterol, 1273mg sodium, 32g carbohydrate, 3g fiber, 27g protein

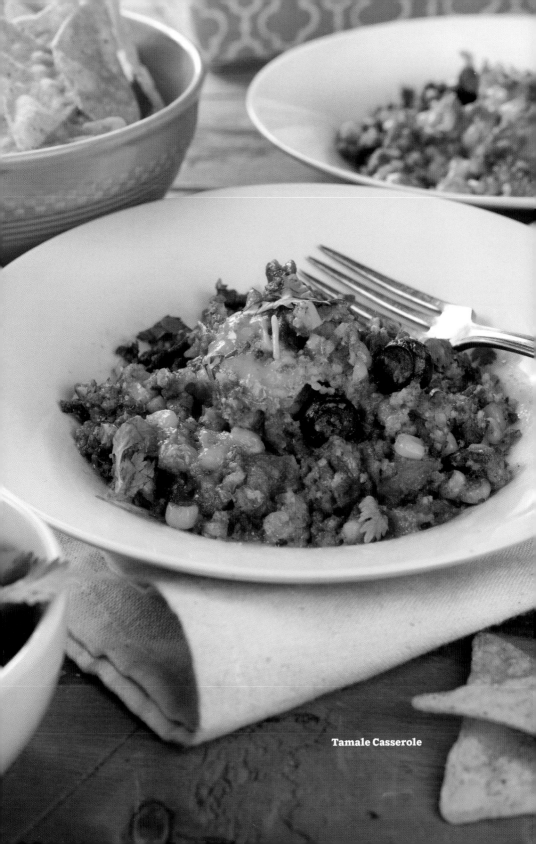

Tamale Casserole

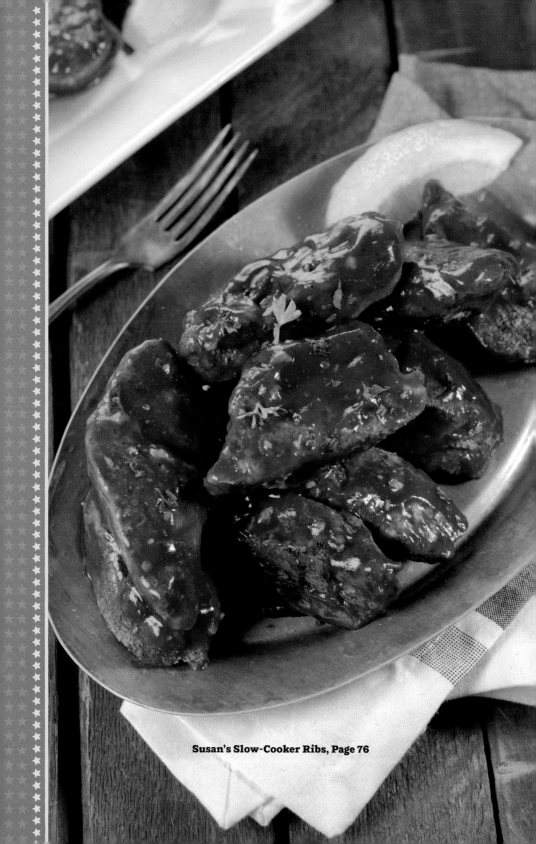

Susan's Slow-Cooker Ribs, Page 76

CHAPTER THREE

Pork

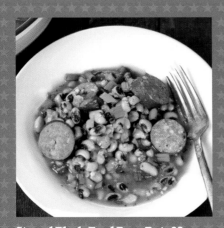

Stewed Black-Eyed Peas, Page 82

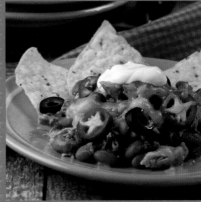

Southwestern Pork Chalupas, Page 70

Nancy Wise, Little Rock, AR

Garlicky Herbed Pork Roast

This is a delicious, hearty roast that serves a crowd. Prep work is a snap, which makes it a great choice when company's coming over for dinner.

Makes 16 servings

4-lb. pork roast
4 cloves garlic, slivered
1 t. dried thyme
1/2 t. dried sage
1/2 t. ground cloves
1 t. salt
1 t. lemon zest
2 T. cold water
2 T. cornstarch

Cut tiny slits into roast with a knife tip; insert garlic slivers. Combine seasonings and zest; rub over roast. Place roast in a slow cooker. Cover and cook on low setting for 7 to 9 hours. or on high setting for 4 to 5 hours. Allow roast to stand 10 to 15 minutes before slicing. Remove and discard garlic pieces. Strain juices into a saucepan over medium heat; bring to a boil. Mix together water and cornstarch until dissolved; gradually add to saucepan. Cook until thickened, about 5 minutes. Serve gravy over sliced pork.

Nutrition Per Serving: 243 calories, 16g total fat, 6g sat fat, 68mg cholesterol, 195mg sodium, 2g carbohydrate, 0g fiber, 23g protein

---

★ LOW-CAL ADD-ON ★ **Pair with mashed sweet potatoes for a 125-calorie side that perfectly complements the fall spices in the roast.**

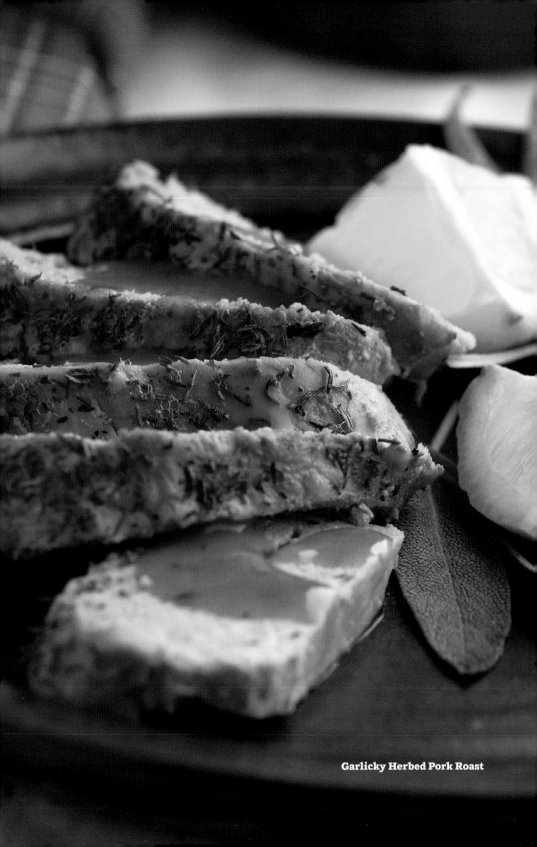

Garlicky Herbed Pork Roast

Ruth Leonard, Columbus OH

Chinese-Style BBQ Pork

We ate this pork roast when we lived in China. Serve with steamed rice and stir-fried veggies like broccoli, carrots and peppers.

Makes 8 servings

2-lb. boneless pork roast
1/4 c. reduced-sodium soy sauce
1/4 c. hoisin sauce
3 T. catsup
3 T. honey
2 t. garlic, minced
2 t. fresh ginger, peeled and grated
1 t. dark sesame oil
1/2 t. Chinese 5-spice powder
1/2 c. chicken broth

Place roast in a large plastic zipping bag and set aside. In a small bowl, whisk together remaining ingredients except broth; pour over roast. Seal bag; refrigerate at least 2 hours, turning occasionally. Place roast in a slow cooker; pour marinade from bag over roast. Cover and cook on low setting for 8 hours. Remove pork from slow cooker; keep warm. Add broth to slow cooker; cover and cook on low setting for 30 minutes, or until thickened. Shred pork with 2 forks and stir into sauce in slow cooker.

Nutrition Per Serving: 300 calories, 17g total fat, 6g sat fat, 69mg cholesterol, 584mg sodium, 13g carbohydrate, 0g fiber, 24g protein

Jody Erdmann, Watertown, WI

Teriyaki Pork Roast

This is my family's spin on one of our take-out favorites...with this recipe we can have it anytime too.

Makes 8 servings

3/4 c. apple juice
2 T. sugar
2 T. reduced-sodium soy sauce
1 T. cider vinegar
1 t. ground ginger
1/4 t. garlic powder
1/8 t. pepper
3-lb. boneless center-cut rolled pork roast
1-1/2 T. cornstarch
3 T. cold water
Garnish: sliced green onions

Combine apple juice, sugar, soy sauce, vinegar and seasonings in a slow cooker; mix well. Add roast, turning to coat; place roast fat-side up. Cover and cook on low setting for 7 to 8 hours. Strain liquid into a small saucepan; bring to a boil. Mix together cornstarch and water in a small bowl; add to boiling liquid. Cook until thickened. Serve gravy over sliced pork; sprinkle with green onions.

Nutrition Per Serving: 236 calories, 6g total fat, 2 sat fat, 106mg cholesterol, 299mg sodium, 11gcarbohydrate, 0g fiber, 35 protein

★ LOW-CAL ADD-ON ★ Serve over 1/2 cup cooked brown rice for an extra 125 calories per serving.

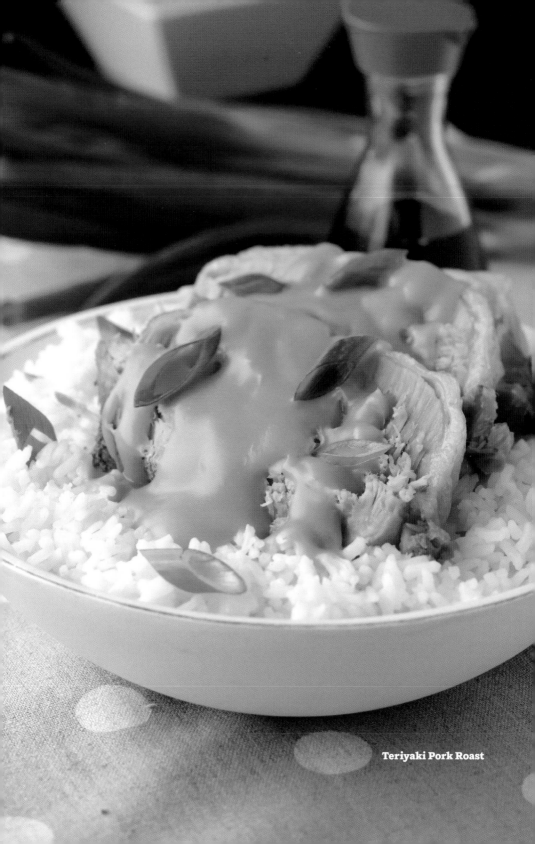

Teriyaki Pork Roast

Carrie Knotts, Kalispell, MT

Easy Pork & Sauerkraut

After several hours of cooking, the flavor of this dish is scrumptious. Use a lager beer for a crisper taste.

Makes 6 servings

1-1/2 lb. boneless pork roast
32-oz. jar low-sodium sauerkraut
12-oz. bottle regular or non-alcoholic beer
1/2 apple, peeled and cored
1 T. garlic, minced
2 t. dill weed
1 t. dry mustard

Combine all ingredients in a slow cooker; stir well. Cover and cook on high setting for one hour. Reduce to low setting and continue cooking for 5 hours, or until pork is cooked through. Discard apple before serving.

Nutrition Per Serving: 210 calories, 5g total fat, 2g sat fat, 71mg cholesterol, 520mg sodium, 15g carbohydrate, 4g fiber, 26g protein

★ LOW-CAL ADD-ON ★ **Serve each portion of pork and sauerkraut over 1/2 cup mashed potatoes for an extra 100 calories.**

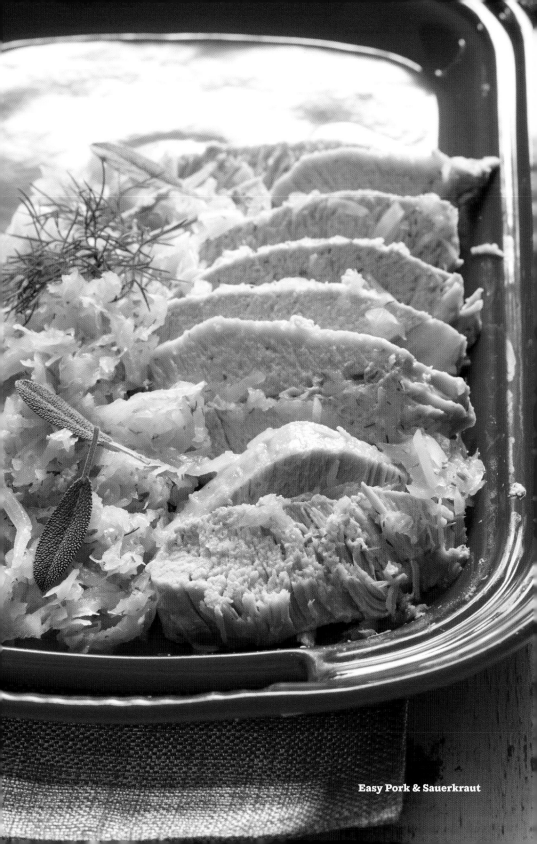

Easy Pork & Sauerkraut

Marion Sundberg, Ramona, CA

Apple Orchard Pork Roast

This roast cooks up so tender...you'll love the apples and vegetables, too.

Makes 8 servings

2-lb. pork shoulder roast, fat trimmed
1 T. olive oil
2 tart apples, peeled, cored and sliced
6 new redskin potatoes
1 onion, coarsely chopped
1 lb. baby carrots
10-3/4 oz. can cream of celery or
   mushroom soup
1 T. Worcestershire sauce to taste
1 t. salt
1 t. pepper

In a skillet over medium heat, brown roast in oil on all sides; place in a slow cooker. Add apples and vegetables; top with remaining ingredients. Cover and cook on low setting for 7 to 8 hours, until roast is cooked through. Arrange sliced pork and vegetables on a platter. Serve with cooking juices, thickened in a saucepan on the stove if necessary.

Nutrition Per Serving: 391 calories, 15g total fat, 5g sat fat, 70mg cholesterol, 657mg sodium, 41g carbohydrate, 7g fiber, 23g protein

Kathleen Hendrick, Alexandria, KY

Savory Slow-Cooked Pork Loin

This is one of my family's favorite recipes...the pork is always tender and delicious.

Makes 8 servings

2-lb. pork loin, quartered
1.2-oz. pkg. brown gravy mix
1 c. water
1 c. apple juice
1/2 c. applesauce
2 t. Worcestershire sauce
1 stalk celery, sliced into 1/2-inch
   pieces
1 onion, chopped
1-1/2 t. seasoned salt
1/2 t. pepper
Optional: 1 T. cornstarch, 1 T. water

Place pork in a slow cooker. In a bowl, combine gravy mix and water; stir until dissolved. Add remaining ingredients except optional cornstarch and water to gravy mixture. Mix well and spoon over pork. Cover and cook on low setting for 8 hours, or until pork is very tender. If liquid in slow cooker needs to be thickened, whisk together cornstarch and one tablespoon water in a cup. Stir into slow cooker during the last 30 minutes of cooking.

Nutrition Per Serving: 233 calories, 12g total fat, 4g sat fat, 64mg cholesterol, 566mg sodium, 9g carbohydrate, 0g fiber, 22g protein

★ SKINNY SECRET ★ To cut extra calories, pour the cooking liquid into a bowl and chill in the refrigerator for a few minutes. Skim the fat off the top and reheat before serving.

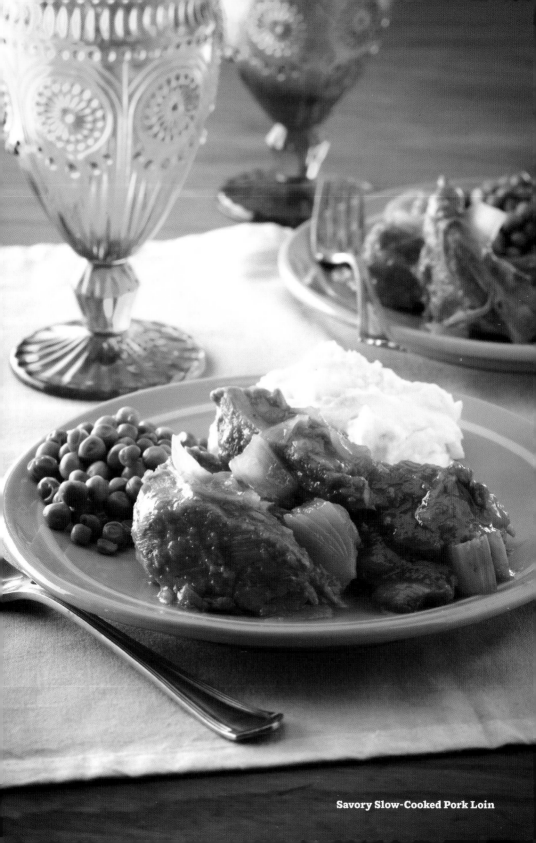

Savory Slow-Cooked Pork Loin

Leslie McMahon, Houston, TX

Pork Loin Roast & Gravy

I started making this dish when my husband and I were just newlyweds. He loves it, and I've continued making it ever since!

Makes 16 servings

4-lb. pork loin end roast, tied with
   kitchen string
2 t. salt
1 t. pepper
1 clove garlic, thinly sliced
2 onions, sliced and divided
1 bay leaf
1 c. hot water
2 T. Worcestershire sauce
2 T. cornstarch
2 T. cold water

Season roast on all sides with salt and pepper. Cut tiny slits into roast with a knife tip; insert thin slices of garlic into slits. Arrange one sliced onion in the bottom of a slow cooker; top with roast. Place remaining sliced onion on top of roast; add remaining ingredients except cornstarch and water. Cover and cook on low setting for 8 to 10 hours, until roast is very tender. Remove roast and onions to a serving platter; discard bay leaf. In a cup, combine cornstarch and water; whisk into juices in slow cooker. Increase heat to high setting and cook gravy for 15 minutes, until thickened. Serve sliced roast and onions drizzled with gravy.

Nutrition Per Serving: 267 calories, 14g total fat, 5g sat fat, 85mg cholesterol, 320mg sodium, 5g carbohydrate, 0g fiber, 30g protein

★ LOW-CAL ADD-ON ★ **Round out the meal with 1/2 cup mashed sweet potatoes and one cup steamed broccoli per serving for an additional 130 calories.**

Arthur Cooper, Indio, CA

Swedish Cabbage Rolls

Comfort food...just like Mom used to make.

Makes 6 servings

12 large cabbage leaves
1 egg, beaten
1/4 c. 2% reduced-fat milk
1/2 c. onion, finely chopped
1 t. salt
1/4 t. pepper
1 lb. ground pork
1 c. cooked rice
8-oz. can tomato sauce
1 T. lemon juice
1 t. Worcestershire sauce
Garnish: sour cream

Cook cabbage leaves in a large kettle of boiling water for 3 to 5 minutes, or until limp; drain well and set aside. Combine egg, milk, onion, salt, pepper, pork and cooked rice; mix well. Place about 1/4 cup meat mixture in the center of each leaf; fold in sides and roll ends over meat. Arrange cabbage rolls in a slow cooker. Combine remaining ingredients except garnish and pour over rolls. Cover and cook on low setting for 7 to 9 hours. Spoon sauce over rolls and garnish with sour cream.

Nutrition Per Serving: 253 calories, 13g total fat, 4g sat fat, 83mg cholesterol, 727mg sodium, 16g carbohydrate, 3g fiber, 17g protein

Trella Ary, Hornbeak, TN

Cabbage & Pork Chops

Sure is good to come home to this meal on a cold and busy day!

Makes 8 servings

4 c. cabbage, shredded
2 apples, peeled, cored and coarsely chopped
1 onion, chopped
1/3 c. brown sugar, packed
1/2 c. cider vinegar
1/2 c. apple juice
1 t. salt, divided
3 lbs. boneless pork chops, fat trimmed
1/4 t. pepper
1 T. olive oil

In a slow cooker, combine cabbage, apples, onion, brown sugar, vinegar, apple juice and 1/2 teaspoon salt. Mix well; spoon into a slow cooker and set aside. Sprinkle pork chops with remaining salt and pepper. Heat oil in a large skillet over medium heat; add pork chops and brown on both sides. Arrange pork chops over cabbage mixture. Cover and cook on low setting for 6 hours, or until pork chops are fork-tender.

Nutrition Per Serving: 357 calories, 13g total fat, 4g sat fat, 93mg cholesterol, 384mg sodium, 22g carbohydrate, 2g fiber, 38g protein

Vickie, Gooseberry Patch

Southwestern Pork Chalupas

You're going to love this zesty dish! I like to serve it with a chopped tomato and avocado salad.

Makes 10 servings

2 15-oz. cans pinto beans, drained and rinsed
4-oz. can chopped green chiles
4 c. water
2 T. chili powder
2 t. ground cumin
1 t. dried oregano
1 t. salt
1 t. pepper to taste
2-lb. pork shoulder roast
9-oz. pkg. multi-grain tortilla chips
Garnish: shredded Mexican-blend cheese, sour cream, salsa, sliced black olives, sliced jalapeño peppers

Combine beans, chiles, water and spices in a large slow cooker; mix well. Add roast; cover and cook on low setting for 4 hours. Remove roast and shred, discarding any bones; return pork to slow cooker. Cover and cook on low setting for an additional 2 to 4 hours, adding more water if necessary. To serve, arrange tortilla chips on serving plates. Spoon pork mixture over chips; garnish as desired.

Nutrition Per Serving: 364 calories, 19g total fat, 5g sat fat, 56mg cholesterol, 611mg sodium, 27g carbohydrate, 4g fiber, 21g protein

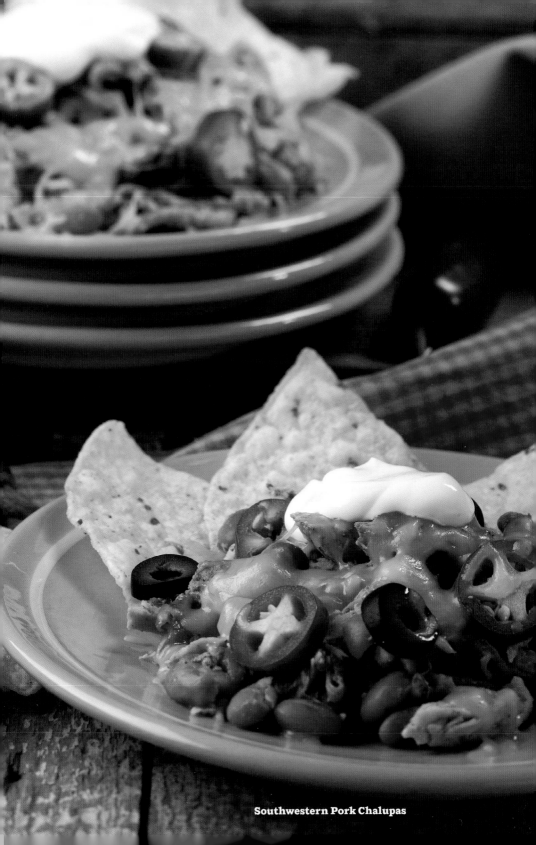

Southwestern Pork Chalupas

Lisa Wagner, Delaware, OH

Savory Pork Carnitas

Try this recipe the next time you're craving tacos or burritos. You can also enjoy it as a main dish, topped with all the garnishes.

Makes 12 servings

3-lb. Boston butt pork roast
1-1/4 oz. pkg. taco seasoning mix
3 cloves garlic, sliced
1 onion, quartered
4-oz. can green chiles, drained
3/4 to 1 c. water
12 6-inch whole wheat flour tortillas
Garnish: shredded lettuce, chopped
   tomatoes, sliced green onions, sour
   cream, lime wedges, fresh cilantro

Place pork roast in a slow cooker; set aside. In a bowl, combine seasoning mix, garlic, onion, chiles and water. Stir to combine and pour over roast. Cover and cook on low setting for 8 to 10 hours, or on high setting for 5 to 6 hours, until tender enough to shred. Spoon shredded pork down the center of tortillas. Roll up and serve with desired garnishes.

Nutrition Per Serving: 354 calories, 18g total fat, 7g sat fat, 96mg cholesterol, 532mg sodium, 17g carbohydrate, 3g fiber, 31g protein

★ LOW-CAL ADD-ON ★ **For only 25 more calories, top each serving with one tablespoon sour cream.**

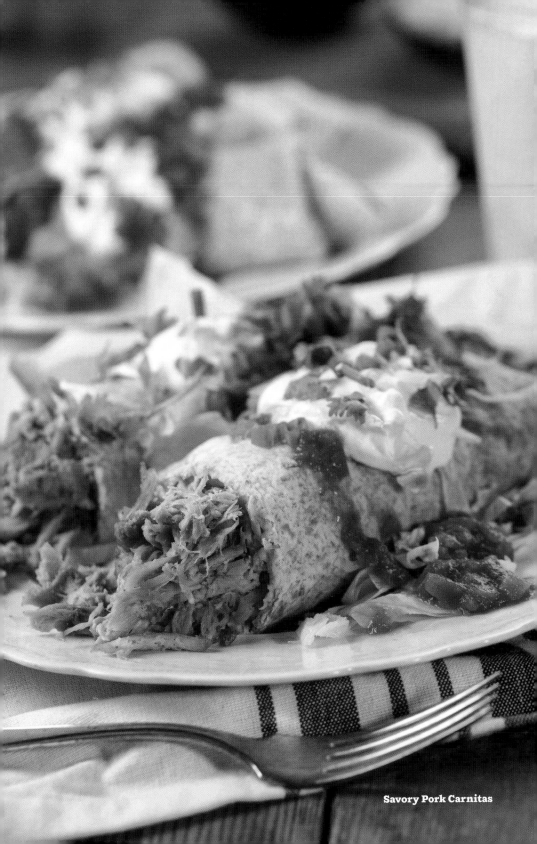

Savory Pork Carnitas

Shannon Molden, Hermiston, OR

Cuban-Style Pork Roast

I love the flavor of this dish...savory and warm, but without a lot of heat. It can be served many different ways and is not only economical, but very tasty too. I like to serve this pork over rice with a side of black beans.

Makes 12 servings

2 T. olive oil
2 t. ground cumin
2 t. dried oregano
2 t. salt
1 t. pepper
1/2 t. red pepper flakes
4 cloves garlic, minced
2 T. lime juice
2 T. orange juice
3-lb. boneless pork shoulder
6 c. cooked brown rice

In a small bowl, mix together oil, seasonings, garlic and juices; set aside. Pierce pork roast all over with a fork; place in a slow cooker. Pour oil mixture over pork; turn to coat well. Cover and cook on low setting for 5 to 6 hours, turning halfway through, until pork is very tender. Remove pork from slow cooker; shred with 2 forks. Return shredded pork to juices in slow cooker; mix well. To serve, spoon pork and some of the juices from slow cooker over rice.

Nutrition Per Serving: 282 calories, 8g total fat, 2g sat fat, 70mg cholesterol, 494mg sodium, 27g carbohydrate, 2g fiber, 26g protein

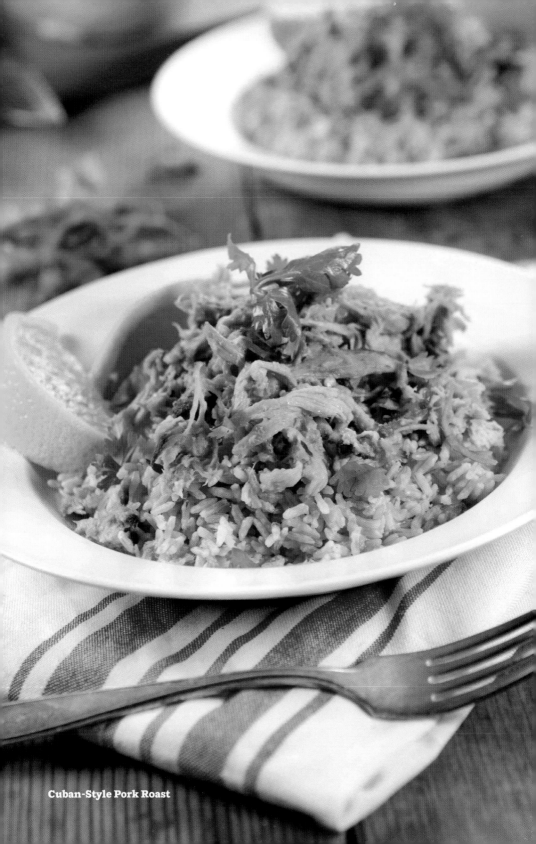

Cuban-Style Pork Roast

Susan Ice, Snohomish, WA

Susan's Slow-Cooker Ribs

You'll love these tender ribs... they're saucy and flavorful.

Makes 8 servings

1 T. onion powder
1 t. red pepper flakes
1/2 t. dry mustard
1/2 t. garlic powder
1/2 t. allspice
1/2 t. cinnamon
3 lbs. boneless pork ribs, sliced into serving-size pieces
1 onion, sliced and divided
1/2 c. water
2 c. low-sodium hickory-flavored barbecue sauce

Combine seasonings in a cup; mix well and rub over ribs. Arrange 1/3 of ribs in a layer in a slow cooker. Place 1/3 of onion slices over top; repeat layering. Pour water over top. Cover and cook on low setting for 8 to 10 hours. Drain and discard liquid from slow cooker. Pour barbecue sauce over ribs. Cover and cook on low setting for an additional one to 2 hours.

Nutrition Per Serving: 398 calories, 20g total fat, 7g sat fat, 123mg cholesterol, 426mg sodium, 23g carbohydrate, 0g fiber, 32g protein

Shelley Turner, Boise ID

Down-Home Beans & Ham

Add a basket of warm corn muffins...yum!

Makes 8 servings

1 lb. dried lima beans
1/2 lb. lean ham or center-cut bacon, diced
10-3/4 oz. can tomato soup
1 c. water
1 onion, chopped
1 green pepper, chopped
1 t. dry mustard
1 t. salt
1 t. pepper

Cover dried beans with water and let soak overnight; drain. Combine beans with remaining ingredients in a slow cooker; mix well. Cover and cook on low setting for 7 to 10 hours, or on high setting for 4 to 5 hours, adding a little more water if needed.

Nutrition Per Serving: 225 calories, 2g total fat, 1g sat fat, 14mg cholesterol, 1084mg sodium, 35g carbohydrate, 11g fiber, 17g protein

★ LOW-CAL ADD-ON ★ A 1-1/2 ounce corn muffin only has 125 calories.

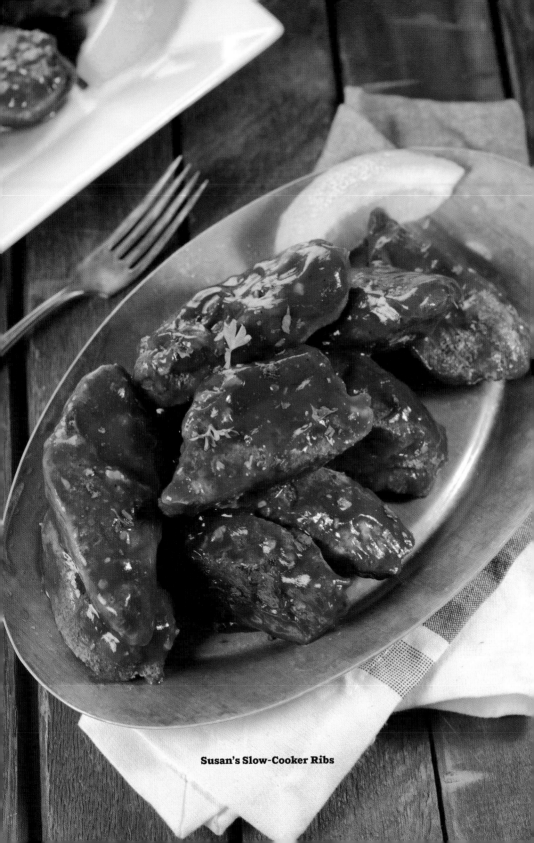

Susan's Slow-Cooker Ribs

Leslie McKinley, Macomb, MO

Mike's Irresistible Italian Chops

My dad is a master at cooking meats, and this is one of his signature dishes! Slice the onions instead of chopping them, if desired.

Makes 5 servings

5 6-oz. pork chops
1-1/2 onions, coarsely chopped
15-oz. can stewed tomatoes
2 T. olive oil
1-1/2 t. Italian seasoning
1-1/2 t. garlic powder
2 t. smoke-flavored cooking sauce
1/4 c. water
2-1/2 c. cooked couscous

Layer pork chops and onions in a slow cooker; add tomatoes with juice and remaining ingredients except couscous. Cover and cook on low setting for 3 to 4 hours, until pork chops are tender. Serve pork chops and sauce from slow cooker over couscous.

Nutrition Per Serving: 380 calories, 11g total fat, 2g sat fat, 95mg cholesterol, 389mg sodium, 26g carbohydrate, 3g fiber, 44g protein

★ SAVVY SWAP ★ We also enjoy these saucy chops over 1/2 cup cooked noodles or rice instead of the couscous.

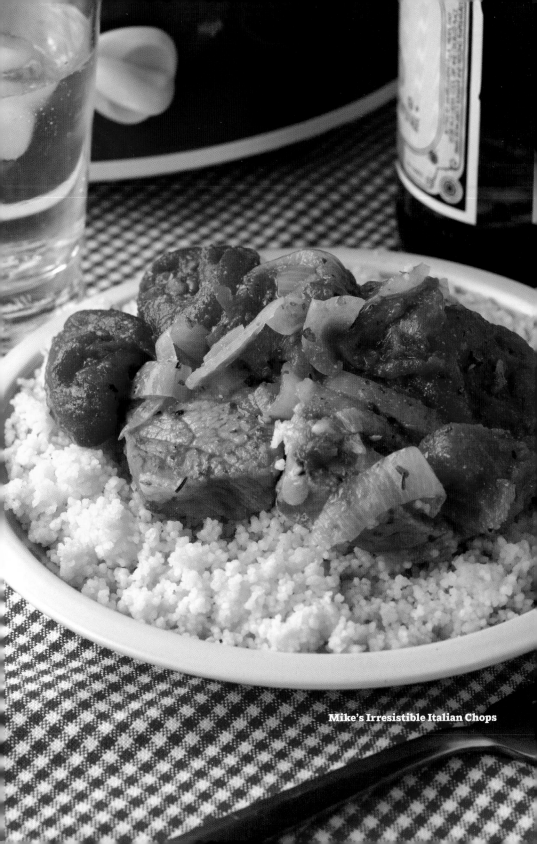

Mike's Irresistible Italian Chops

Marsha Baker, Pioneer, OH

Hearty Red Beans & Rice

For an added hit of heat, serve with your favorite hot sauce.

Makes 8 servings

1 lb. dried kidney beans
2 T. oil
1 onion, chopped
3 stalks celery, chopped
1 green pepper, chopped
2 cloves garlic, minced
3 c. water
2-2/3 c. low-sodium beef broth
1/2 t. red pepper flakes
1 meaty ham bone
4 c. cooked brown rice
Garnish: chopped green onions

Soak beans overnight in enough water to cover; drain and set aside. In a large skillet, heat oil over medium-high heat. Add onion, celery, green pepper and garlic; sauté until onion is translucent, 5 to 6 minutes. Place in a slow cooker along with drained beans, water, broth and red pepper flakes. Add ham bone and push down into mixture. Cover and cook on low setting for 10 hours. Remove ham bone; dice meat and return to slow cooker. Serve beans spooned over hot cooked rice in bowls. Garnish with green onions.

Nutrition Per Serving: 362 calories, 9g total fat, 2g sat fat, 28mg cholesterol, 417mg sodium, 46g carbohydrate, 9g fiber, 24g protein

Lisa Quick, Clarksburg, MD

Scalloped Potatoes & Ham

This is an incredibly filling main dish recipe. Serve it with a side of cooked greens to complete the meal.

Makes 8 servings

8 potatoes, peeled and sliced
1 c. cooked lean ham, diced
1 small onion, diced
1/2 c. reduced-fat shredded Cheddar cheese
10-3/4 oz. can cream of chicken soup

In a slow cooker, layer each ingredient in the order given, spreading soup over top. Do not stir. Cover and cook on low setting for 8 to 10 hours, or on high setting for 5 hours.

Nutrition Per Serving: 353 calories, 7g total fat, 2g sat fat, 25mg cholesterol, 570mg sodium, 62g carbohydrate, 5g fiber, 11g protein

---

★ SAVVY SWAP ★ **Use smoked turkey sausage instead of the ham.**

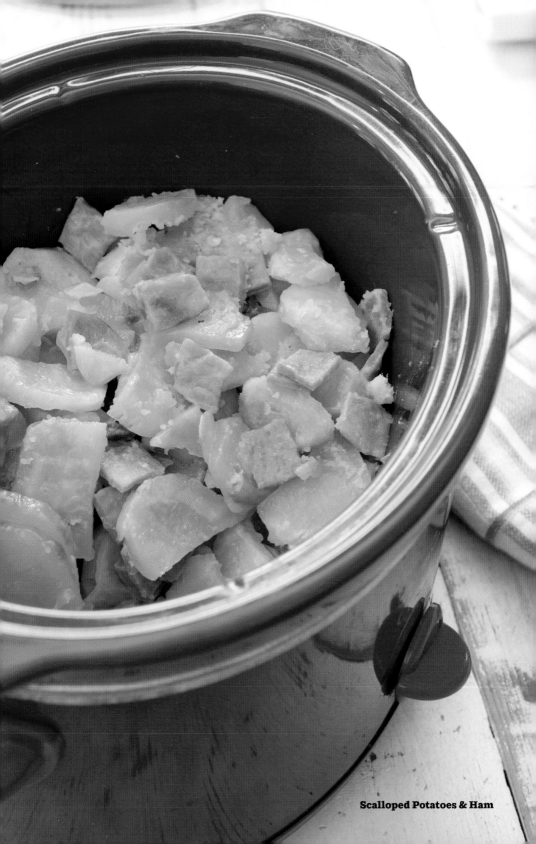

Scalloped Potatoes & Ham

Leslie Stimel, Columbus, OH

Stewed Black-Eyed Peas

Andouille is a spicy sausage from Louisiana. Substitute another spicy smoked sausage, if you like.

Makes 10 servings

1 lb. dried black-eyed peas
1 lb. andouille pork sausage, cut into
    1/4-inch slices
1 c. yellow onion, chopped
1/2 t. salt
2 T. hot pepper sauce
5 cloves garlic, pressed
4 bay leaves
1 t. dried thyme
1 t. dried parsley
8 c. chicken broth

Combine all ingredients in a slow cooker; cover and cook on low setting for 5 to 6 hours. Discard bay leaves before serving.

Nutrition Per Serving: 261 calories, 7g total fat, 2g sat fat, 31mg cholesterol, 1300mg sodium, 31g carbohydrate, 7g fiber, 19g protein

★ LOW-CAL ADD-ON ★ Make this recipe a one-dish meal by and serve over 1/2 cup hot cooked rice for 120 more calories.

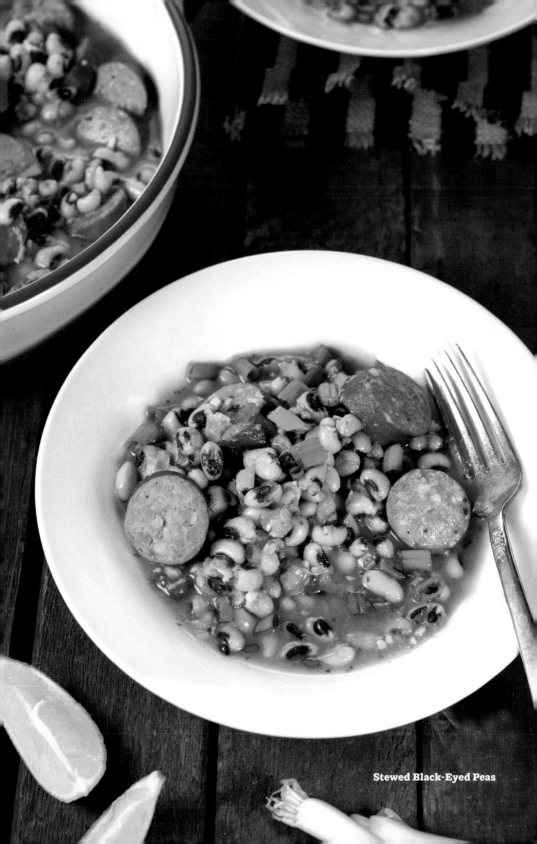

Stewed Black-Eyed Peas

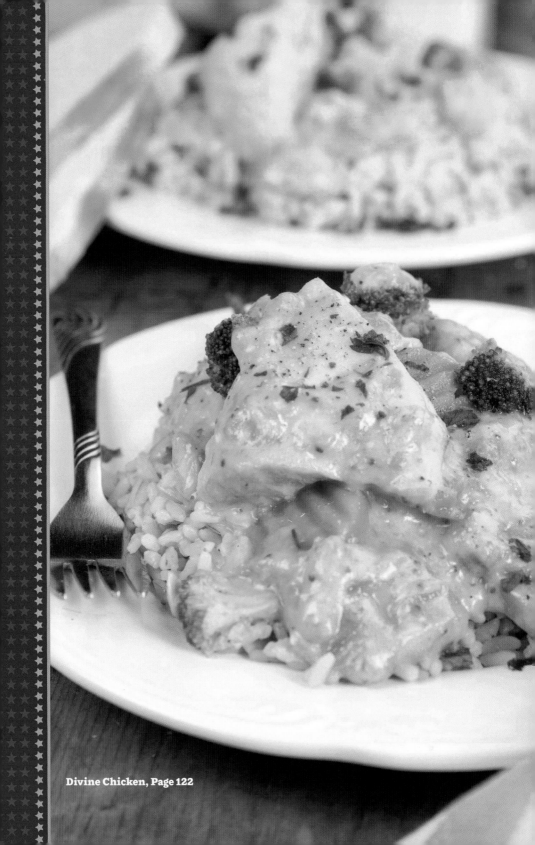

Divine Chicken, Page 122

CHAPTER FOUR

Poultry

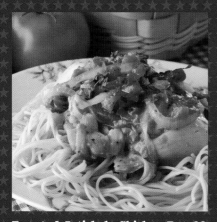

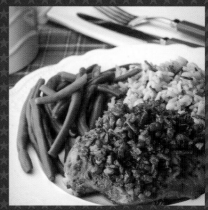

Tomato & Artichoke Chicken, Page 96   **Maple Praline Chicken, Page 104**

Rhonda Reeder, Ellicott City, MD

Slow-Cooker Chicken & Dumplings

With a slow cooker, you can serve your family a homestyle dinner even after a busy day away from home.

Makes 8 servings

1-1/2 lbs. boneless, skinless chicken
   breasts, cubed
1 T. olive oil
2 potatoes, peeled and cubed
2 c. baby carrots
2 stalks celery, sliced
10-3/4 oz. can low-sodium cream of
   chicken soup
1 c. water
1 c. 2% reduced-fat milk
1 t. dried thyme
1/4 t. pepper
2 c. reduced-fat biscuit baking mix
2/3 c. whole milk

In a skillet over medium heat, cook chicken in oil just until golden on all sides. Place chicken, potatoes, carrots and celery in a slow cooker; set aside. In a bowl, combine soup, water, reduced-fat milk, thyme and pepper; pour over chicken mixture. Cover and cook on low setting for 7 to 8 hours, until chicken is tender. Mix together baking mix and whole milk; drop into slow cooker by large spoonfuls. Cover and cook on high setting for 30 minutes, or until dumplings are cooked in center.

Nutrition Per Serving: 321 calories, 7g total fat, 1g sat fat, 55mg cholesterol, 508mg sodium, 40g carbohydrate, 2g fiber, 26g protein

---

★ SKINNY SECRET ★ A bit of 2% reduced-fat milk combined with the canned soup gives the chicken mixture the right amount of creaminess without the need to add high-calorie cream or whole milk.

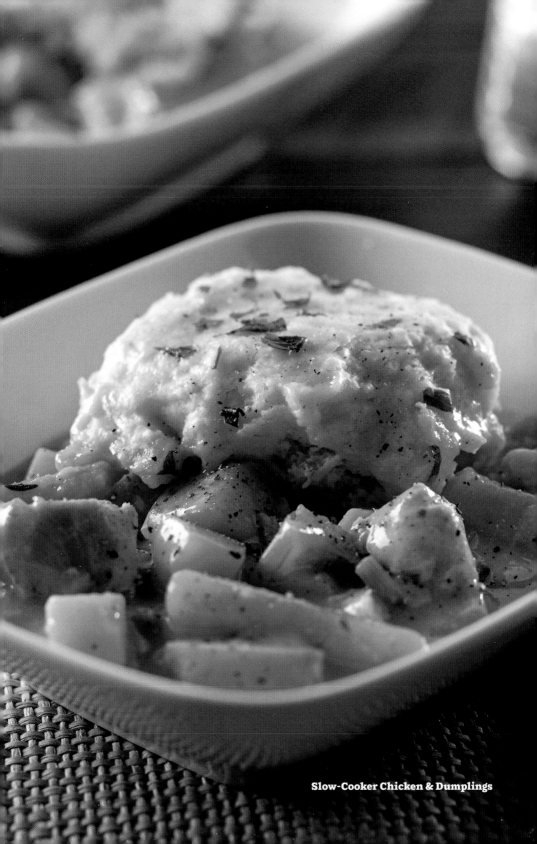

Slow-Cooker Chicken & Dumplings

Shirley Howie, Foxboro, MA

Herbed Chicken & Wild Rice

This savory recipe is quick & easy to prepare. It has become one of my favorites for the slow cooker.

Makes 6 servings

6-oz. pkg. long grain and wild rice mix
6 6-oz. boneless, skinless chicken
  breasts
1 T. olive oil
1 t. butter
1/2 lb. sliced mushrooms
10-3/4 oz. can cream of chicken soup
1-1/4 c. water
3 slices center-cut bacon, crisply
  cooked and crumbled, or 3 T.
  bacon bits
1 t. dried parsley
1/2 t. dried thyme
1/2 t. dried basil

Place uncooked rice in a 5-quart slow cooker; set aside seasoning packet. In a large skillet over medium heat, brown chicken breasts in oil and butter on both sides. Add chicken to slow cooker. In the same skillet, sauté mushrooms until tender; spoon over chicken. In a small bowl, whisk together soup, water, bacon, herbs and contents of seasoning packet. Pour over mushrooms. Cover and cook on low setting for 4 hours, or until chicken juices run clear when pierced.

Nutrition Per Serving: 228 calories, 9g total fat, 2g sat fat, 28mg cholesterol, 721mg sodium, 25g carbohydrate, 3g fiber, 12g protein

★ SAVVY SWAP ★ Try this easy substitution for canned cream soups. In a bowl, combine one tablespoon softened butter, 3 tablespoons flour, 1/2 cup 1% low-fat milk, 1/2 cup chicken broth and salt and pepper to taste. Blend well and use as you would one 10-3/4 ounce can cream soup.

Kathy Kyler, Norman, OK

Cozy Chicken & Noodles

I got this recipe from a co-worker several years ago. It is my husband's favorite meal in cold weather, and it reheats well. Serve with some crusty bread to mop up the tasty sauce...it will chase away the winter chills!

Makes 6 servings

10-3/4 oz. can cream of chicken soup
4 c. low-sodium chicken broth
3 carrots, peeled and chopped
3 stalks celery, chopped
1/4 c. butter, sliced
1 t. garlic powder
pepper to taste
1 bay leaf
4 6-oz. boneless, skinless chicken breasts
8-oz. pkg. wide egg noodles, uncooked

In a slow cooker, stir together soup, broth, vegetables, butter and seasonings. Push chicken down into mixture. Cover and cook on low setting for 6 to 8 hours. About 30 minutes before serving, turn slow cooker to high setting. Stir uncooked noodles into mixture in slow cooker. Cover and cook until noodles are tender, 10 to 15 minutes. At serving time, discard bay leaf. Remove chicken; cool slightly and shred, then stir back into noodle mixture. To serve, ladle into bowls.

Nutrition Per Serving: 323 calories, 14g total fat, 6g sat fat, 114mg cholesterol, 552mg sodium, 17g carbohydrate, 2g fiber, 30g protein

★ SAVVY SWAP ★ **Sub boneless, skinless chicken thighs for chicken breasts.**

Dina Willard, Abingdon, MD

Creamy Dreamy Chicken

I love to feed my family delicious meals to warm their tummies and their hearts. It's especially nice to know that at the end of a long day, dinner is ready. We can relax and share our stories of the day.

Makes 6 servings

6 4-oz. boneless, skinless chicken
   thighs
2-1/2 lbs. new redskin potatoes or
   Yukon Gold potatoes, halved
1/4 t. salt
1/2 t. pepper
10-oz. pkg. frozen carrots, thawed
1/2 c. green onions, thinly sliced
1-lb. bunch asparagus, trimmed and
   cut into thirds
2 10-3/4 oz. cans cream of mushroom
   soup
1/2 c. unsweetened almond milk or
   1% low-fat milk

In a slow cooker, layer chicken and potatoes; sprinkle with salt and pepper. Add carrots and green onions, mixing gently; place asparagus on top. Whisk together soup and milk in a bowl; pour over top. Cover and cook on low setting for 7 to 8 hours.

Nutrition Per Serving: 391 calories, 10g total fat, 2g sat fat, 90mg cholesterol, 994mg sodium, 45g carbohydrate, 7g fiber, 30g protein

★ LOW-CAL ADD-ON ★ A crisp green salad goes well with this dish. For a zippy homemade citrus dressing, shake up 1/2 cup olive oil, 1/2 cup lemon or orange juice and a tablespoon of Dijon mustard in a small jar and chill. Two tablespoons dressing has 60 calories.

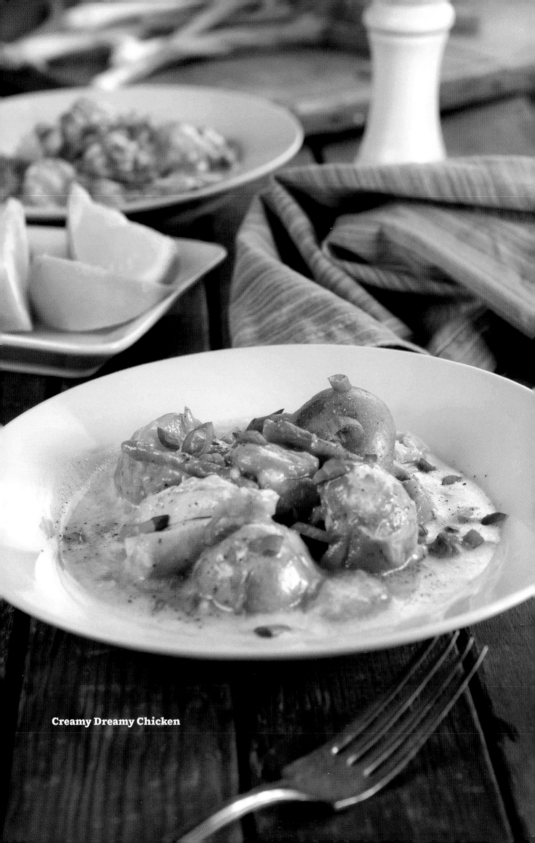

Creamy Dreamy Chicken

Amy Bradsher, Roxboro, NC

Caribbean Chicken & Veggies

I love to serve meals made from scratch, but they can be pretty time-consuming. This recipe is super-simple and cooks on its own, requiring little attention from me. Best of all, my kids love it!

Makes 6 servings

1 lb. boneless, skinless
   chicken tenders
1 c. canned diced pineapple with juice
1 onion, coarsely chopped
1 green pepper, coarsely chopped
3/4 c. Caribbean-style marinade
1-1/2 c. canned black beans, drained
1 lb. broccoli, cut into bite-size
   flowerets
3 c. cooked brown rice

Combine chicken, pineapple with juice, onion, green pepper and marinade in a slow cooker. Cover and cook on low setting for 4 to 5 hours, until chicken is nearly cooked. Add black beans and broccoli. Cover and continue cooking for one hour, or until broccoli is tender. Serve chicken mixture over cooked rice.

Nutrition Per Serving: 385 calories, 4g total fat, 1g sat fat, 55mg cholesterol, 1162mg sodium, 63g carbohydrate, 8g fiber, 26g protein.

Anna McMaster, Portland, OR

Orange-Glazed Chicken

Sweet and delicious.

Makes 6 servings

6-oz. can frozen orange juice
   concentrate, thawed
1 onion, diced
1 clove garlic, minced
1/2 t. dried rosemary
6 6-oz. boneless, skinless chicken
   breasts
1 t. salt
1 t. pepper
1/4 c. cold water
2 T. cornstarch

Combine orange juice, onion, garlic and rosemary in a plastic zipping bag. Add chicken to bag and toss to coat; place chicken in a lightly greased slow cooker. Pour remaining juice mixture over chicken; add salt and pepper. Cover and cook on low setting for 7 to 9 hours. Remove chicken from slow cooker; cover and keep warm. Mix together water and cornstarch; stir into juices in slow cooker. Partially cover slow cooker; cook on high setting until thick and bubbly, about 15 to 30 minutes. To serve, spoon sauce over chicken.

Nutrition Per Serving: 264 calories, 5g total fat, 1g sat fat, 124mg cholesterol, 473mg sodium, 14g carbohydrate, 1g fiber, 39g protein

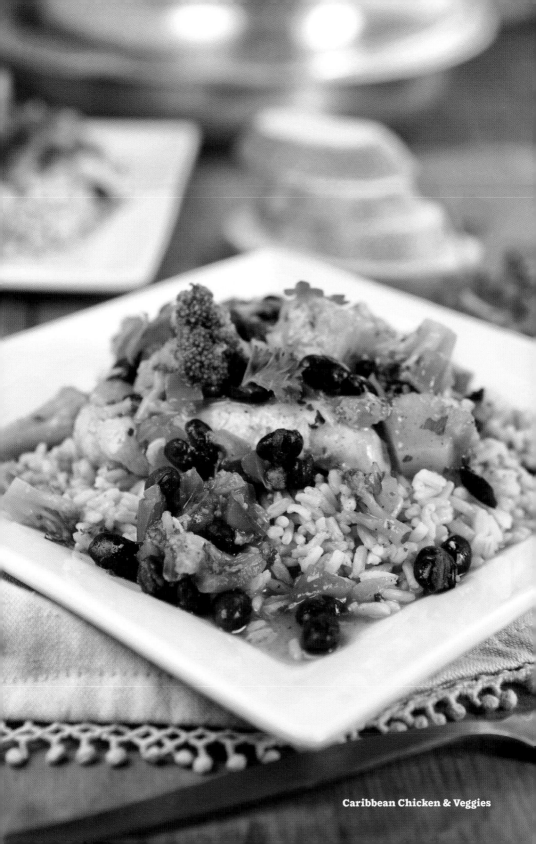

Caribbean Chicken & Veggies

Diane Tracy, Lake Mary, FL

Chicken Parmigiana

This is incredibly delicious...so tender you won't need a knife!

Makes 6 servings

1 egg
3/4 c. 1% low-fat milk
1/2 t. salt
1/2 t. pepper
3/4 c. Italian-seasoned dry bread crumbs
3 6-oz. boneless, skinless chicken breasts, cut in half
1 T. olive oil
26-oz. jar spaghetti sauce, divided
3/4 c. shredded part-skim mozzarella cheese
3 c. cooked spaghetti

Beat together egg and milk in a deep bowl. Add salt and pepper; set aside. Place bread crumbs in a shallow bowl. Dip chicken breasts into egg mixture; coat with crumb mixture. Spray both sides of chicken with non-stick vegetable cooking spray. Heat oil in a skillet over medium heat; cook chicken just until golden on both sides. Add one cup sauce to the bottom of a slow cooker; top with chicken. Spoon remaining sauce over chicken. Cover and cook on low setting for 6 to 8 hours. About 15 minutes before serving, sprinkle cheese over top; cover until melted. Serve chicken and sauce over cooked spaghetti.

Nutrition Per Serving: 379 calories, 12g total fat, 3g sat fat, 107mg cholesterol, 1023mg sodium, 37g carbohydrate, 4g fiber, 31g protein

★ SKINNY SECRET ★ **A smaller portion of both the chicken and the pasta allows for the dish's signature cheesy mozzarella topping.**

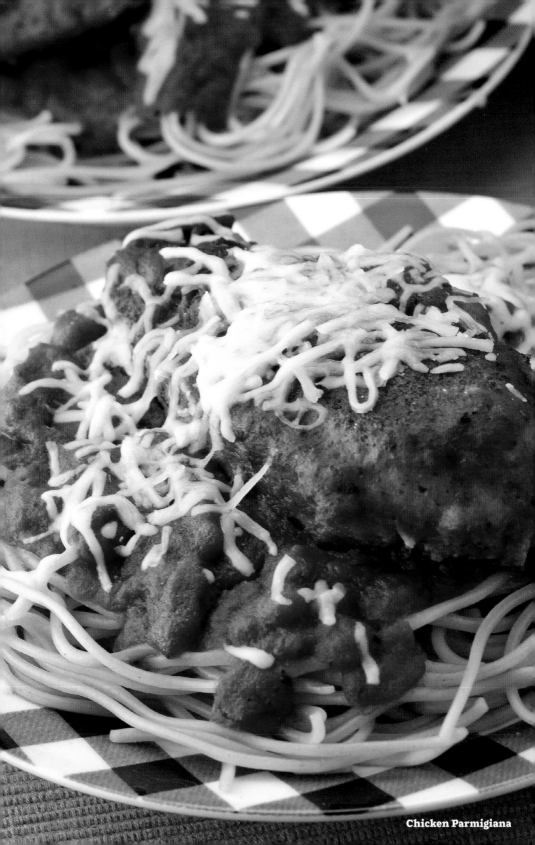

Chicken Parmigiana

Rachel Boyd, Defiance, OH

Tomato & Artichoke Chicken

This is one of the best summer recipes I've tried. The flavor of the artichokes pairs really well with the tomatoes!

Makes 4 servings

4 6-oz. boneless, skinless chicken
   breasts
3 T. Italian salad dressing
1 t. Italian seasoning
1/2 onion, very thinly sliced
4 cloves garlic, minced
14-1/2 oz. can diced tomatoes, drained
14-oz. can quartered artichoke
   hearts, drained
2 to 3 T. dried parsley
2 c. cooked spaghetti

Place chicken in a slow cooker. Combine remaining ingredients except spaghetti; spoon over chicken. Cover and cook on low setting for 4 to 5 hours, until chicken juices run clear. To serve, spoon chicken mixture over cooked spaghetti.

Nutrition Per Serving: 283 calories, 7g total fat, 1g sat fat, 124mg cholesterol, 534mg sodium, 12g carbohydrate, 2g fiber, 41g protein

Jackie Smulski, Lyons, IL

Classic Chicken Cacciatore

Try this rich saucy stew served over rice or thin spaghetti too.

Makes 6 servings

2 T. olive oil
1 lb. boneless, skinless chicken
   breasts, cut into strips
1/2 c. all-purpose flour
pepper to taste
1/2 c. white wine or chicken broth,
   divided
1 onion, chopped
1 green pepper, chopped
2 cloves garlic, minced
1/2 t. dried oregano
1/2 t. dried basil
2 T. fresh Italian parsley, chopped
2 14-oz. cans diced Italian tomatoes
14-oz. jar Italian pasta sauce with
   vegetables
8-oz. pkg. mushrooms, chopped
6-oz. pkg. broad egg noodles, cooked
Garnish: grated Parmesan cheese

Heat olive oil in a slow cooker on high setting. Coat chicken in flour and pepper; add to slow cooker. Cover and cook on high setting for 1-1/2 to 2 hours, until chicken is no longer pink. Stir in 1/4 cup wine or broth. Add onion, green pepper, garlic and herbs; cook until onion is tender. Add tomatoes with juice, pasta sauce and mushrooms; cover and bring to a slow boil, about 30 minutes to one hour. Serve chicken and sauce over cooked noodles; sprinkle with Parmesan cheese.

Nutrition Per Serving: 391 calories, 9g total fat, 2g sat fat, 90mg cholesterol, 617mg sodium, 47g carbohydrate, 6g fiber, 26g protein

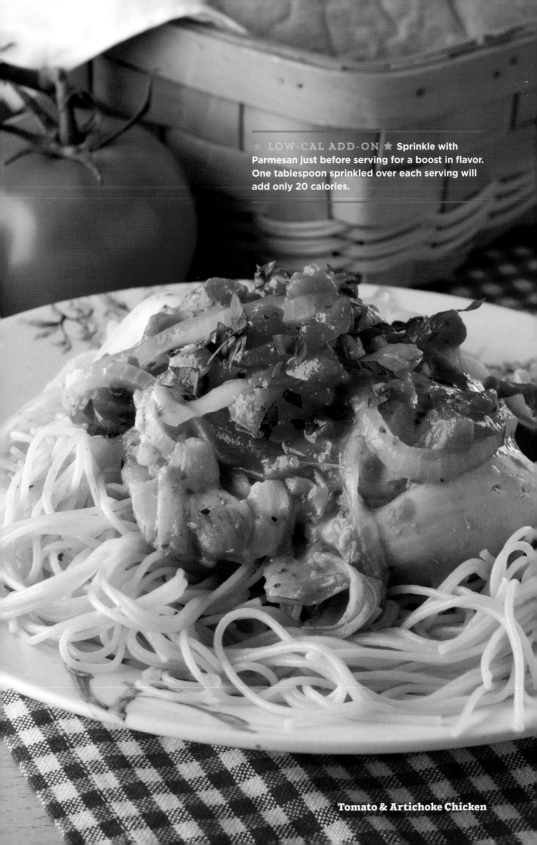

★ LOW·CAL ADD·ON ★ Sprinkle with Parmesan just before serving for a boost in flavor. One tablespoon sprinkled over each serving will add only 20 calories.

Tomato & Artichoke Chicken

Darrell Lawrey, Kissimmee, FL

Chicken & Sausage Paella

Your friends will think you really worked hard on this wonderful dish... we won't tell them otherwise!

Makes 6 servings

2 lbs. boneless, skinless chicken thighs, cubed
1 T. oil
1/2 lb. smoked turkey sausage links, cut into chunks
1 onion, sliced
3 cloves garlic, minced
2 t. dried thyme
1/2 t. pepper
1/8 t. dried saffron or turmeric
14-1/2 oz. can low-sodium chicken broth
1/2 c. water
14-1/2 oz. can diced tomatoes, drained
2 yellow and/or green peppers, thinly sliced
1 c. frozen green peas, thawed
3 c. cooked yellow or white rice

In a large skillet over medium heat, cook chicken in oil until golden on all sides; drain. Place chicken in a large slow cooker; add sausage and onion. Sprinkle with garlic and seasonings. Pour broth and water over all. Cover and cook on low setting for 7 to 8 hours, or on high setting for 3-1/2 to 4 hours. About 15 to 20 minutes before serving, stir in tomatoes, peppers and peas. Cover and cook on low setting until vegetables are tender. Serve mixture ladled over cooked rice.

Nutrition Per Serving: 357 calories, 7g total fat, 1g sat fat, 122mg cholesterol, 708mg sodium, 35g carbohydrate, 4g fiber, 37g protein

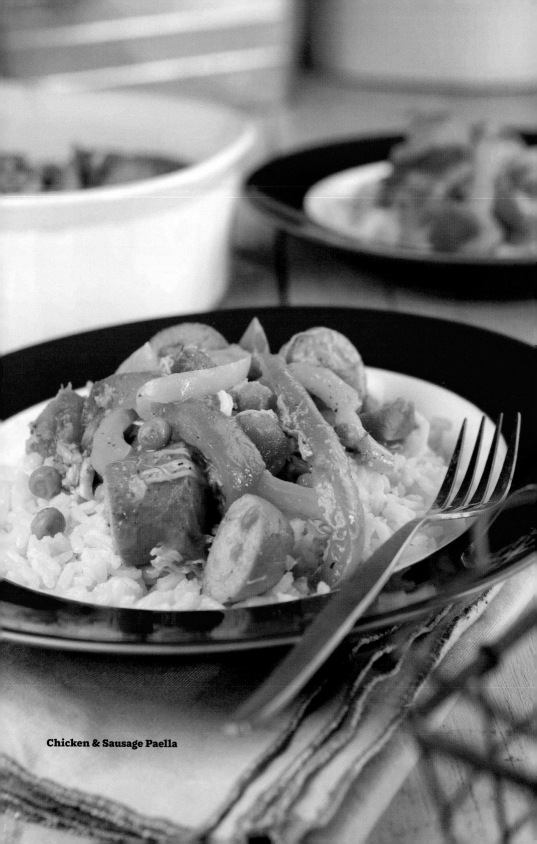

Chicken & Sausage Paella

Valarie Dennard, Palatka, FL

Rosemary & Red Pepper Chicken

An elegant main dish that's so easy to prepare.

Makes 8 servings

1 onion, thinly sliced
1 red pepper, thinly sliced
4 cloves garlic, minced
2 t. dried rosemary
1/2 t. dried oregano
1/2 lb. lean Italian turkey sausage, casings removed
8 6-oz. boneless, skinless chicken breasts
1/4 t. pepper
1/4 c. dry vermouth or low-sodium chicken broth
2 T. cold water
1-1/2 T. cornstarch
3/4 t. salt
Optional: 1/4 c. fresh parsley, chopped
4 c. cooked fettuccine

Combine onion, red pepper, garlic and herbs in a slow cooker. Crumble sausage over top. Arrange chicken over sausage; sprinkle with pepper. Pour in vermouth or broth; cover and cook on low setting for 5 to 7 hours. Transfer chicken to a platter; cover to keep warm. In a small bowl, stir together water and cornstarch. Stir into cooking liquid in slow cooker. Increase heat to high setting; cover and cook until sauce is thickened, stirring 2 to 3 times, about 10 minutes. Sprinkle with salt. Spoon sauce over chicken; sprinkle with chopped parsley, if desired. Serve with cooked fettuccine.

Nutrition Per Serving: 349 calories, 7g total fat, 2g sat fat, 140mg cholesterol, 528mg sodium, 20g carbohydrate, 1g fiber, 46g protein

Sandra Monroe, Preston, MD

Chicken Cacciatore with Zucchini

My husband loves this meal. It's so simple to put together and a good way to use fresh summer vegetables.

Makes 4 servings

1 lb. boneless, skinless chicken breasts
26-oz. jar chunky garden-style pasta sauce
1 zucchini, chopped
1 green pepper, chopped
1 c. onion, chopped
2 c. cooked wide egg noodles or spaghetti
Garnish: grated Parmesan cheese

Spray a slow cooker with non-stick vegetable spray. Add chicken breasts; pour pasta sauce over chicken. Top with vegetables. Cover and cook on low setting for 6 to 8 hours. Serve chicken with sauce mixture from slow cooker, spooned over cooked noodles or spaghetti. Garnish with cheese.

Nutrition Per Serving: 351 calories, 6g total fat, 1g sat fat, 106mg cholesterol, 499mg sodium, 42g carbohydrate, 6g fiber, 33g protein

★ LOW-CAL ADD-ON ★ Try this flavorful salad alongside a rich-tasting main dish. Toss together mixed greens, cherry tomatoes and thinly sliced red onion in a salad bowl. Whisk together 1/4 cup each of balsamic vinegar and olive oil, then drizzle over salad.

Angela Couillard, Lakeville, MN

Sausage-Stuffed Squash

Sweet, savory and so tender! This tasty squash is a welcome addition to a holiday supper, or serve it as a simple weeknight meal.

Makes 4 servings

12-oz. pkg. smoked turkey sausage, diced
1/3 c. dark brown sugar, packed
1/4 t. dried sage
2 acorn squash, halved and seeded
1 c. water

In a bowl, mix together sausage, brown sugar and sage; toss to mix well. Fill squash halves heaping full with sausage mixture; wrap each stuffed half with aluminum foil. Pour water into a large slow cooker; place wrapped squash halves in slow cooker, stacking if necessary. Cover and cook on low setting for 6 to 8 hours, until squash is fork-tender.

Nutrition Per Serving: 349 calories, 10g fat, 2g sat fat, 90mg cholesterol, 708mg sodium, 41g carbohydrate, 3g fiber, 25g protein

★ LOW-CAL ADD-ON ★ Make a fresh-tasting, 50-calorie side dish to serve 6. Combine 3 to 4 sliced zucchini, 1/2 teaspoon minced garlic and a tablespoon of chopped fresh basil. Sauté in a tablespoon of olive oil until tender.

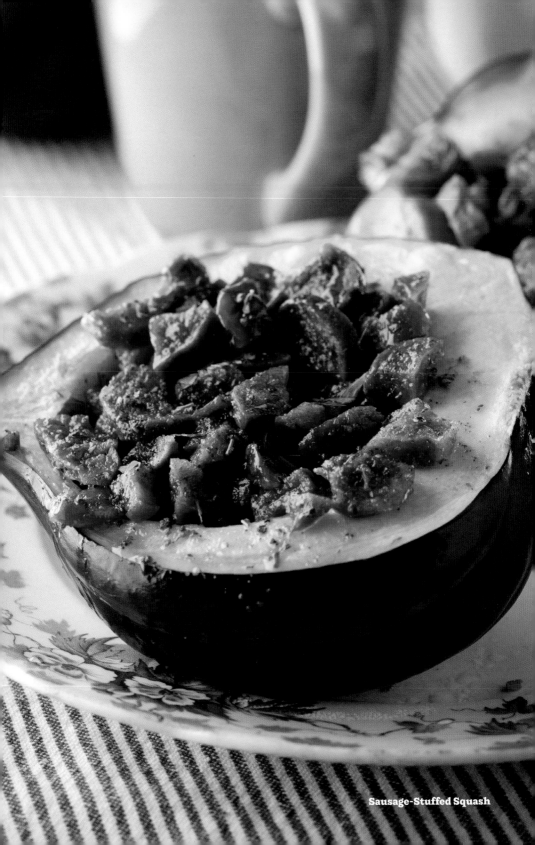

Sausage-Stuffed Squash

Diane Stout, Zeeland, MI

Chicken Italiano

Full of flavor! Serve over
thin spaghetti.

Makes 6 servings

14-1/2 oz. can diced tomatoes, drained
7-oz. can sliced mushrooms, drained
2-1/2 oz. can sliced black olives,
   drained
1/2 c. onion, chopped
1/2 c. green pepper, diced
3 T. tomato paste
2 T. capers
2 T. olive oil
1 T. garlic, minced
1/2 t. salt
1 t. pepper
1/2 t. dried oregano
Optional: 2 T. red wine
2 lbs. boneless, skinless chicken
   thighs

Combine all ingredients except
chicken in a slow cooker; mix well.
Add chicken and stir to coat. Cover
and cook on low setting for 7 to
8 hours, until chicken is tender.

Nutrition Per Serving: 257 calories, 11g
total fat, 2g sat fat, 121mg cholesterol,
657mg sodium, 8g carbohydrate, 2g fiber,
32g protein

Jill Valentine, Jackson, TN

Maple Praline Chicken

I have a neighbor who bottles his
own maple syrup, and it really makes
this dish taste wonderful...so sweet
and flavorful!

Makes 6 servings

6 6-oz. boneless, skinless chicken
   breasts
1 T. Cajun seasoning
2 T. butter
1/3 c. maple syrup
1-1/2 T. brown sugar, packed
1/2 c. chopped pecans
6-oz. pkg. long-grain and wild rice,
   cooked

Sprinkle chicken with Cajun
seasoning. In a skillet over
medium-high heat, cook chicken
in butter until golden. Arrange
chicken in a slow cooker. In a bowl,
mix together syrup, brown sugar and
pecans; spoon over chicken. Cover
and cook on low setting for 6 to
8 hours. Serve chicken with
cooked rice.

Nutrition Per Serving: 397 calories, 13g
total fat, 4g sat fat, 93mg cholesterol,
728mg sodium, 40g carbohydrate, 1g fiber,
29g protein

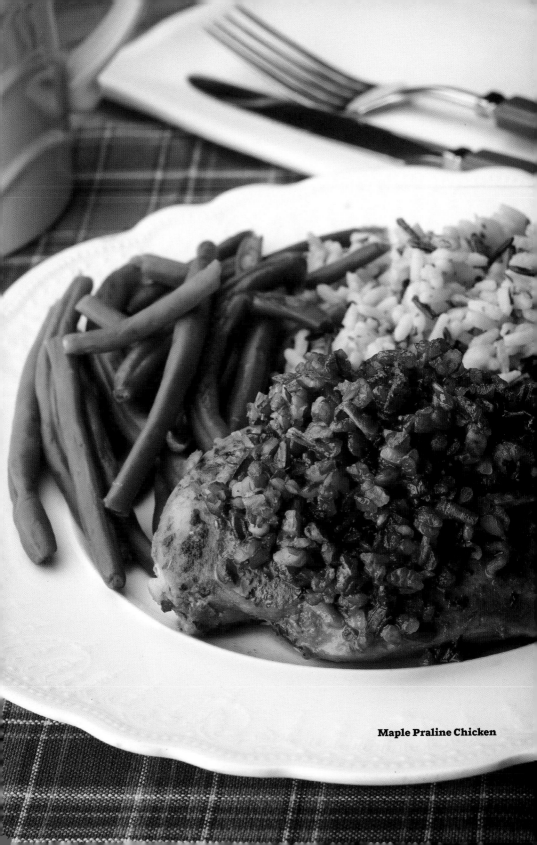

Maple Praline Chicken

Dawn Morgan, Glendora, CA

California Chicken Tacos

We spoon the chicken mixture into crunchy taco shells, but in a pinch you can serve it in flour tortillas instead.

Makes 6 servings

1 lb. boneless, skinless chicken
  breasts
1-1/4 oz. pkg. taco seasoning mix
16-oz. jar favorite salsa
12 corn taco shells
Garnish: shredded lettuce, diced
  tomatoes, sour cream, shredded
  Cheddar cheese

Combine all ingredients except taco shells and garnish. Cover and cook on low setting for 6 to 8 hours, or on high setting for 4 hours. Shred chicken and spoon into taco shells; garnish as desired.

Nutrition Per Serving: 224 calories, 7g total fat, 2g sat fat, 55mg cholesterol, 1138mg sodium, 21g carbohydrate, 3g fiber, 20g protein

★ LOW-CAL ADD-ON ★ For only an extra 15 calories per serving, top each taco with 1/2 tablespoon reduced-fat sour cream and one tablespoon fresh salsa.

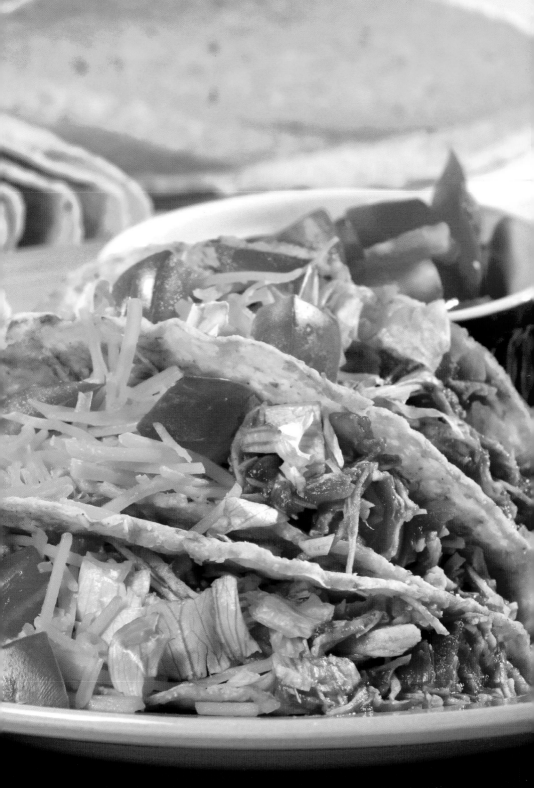

California Chicken Tacos

Katie Foster, Indianola, NE

Spicy Mideastern Turkey

So good...they'll be coming back for seconds!

Makes 6 servings

1-1/2 lbs. boneless, skinless turkey
   tenderloins
1 green pepper, sliced
1-1/4 c. low-sodium chicken broth,
   divided
1/4 c. low-sodium soy sauce
2 cloves garlic, minced
3/4 t. red pepper flakes
2 T. cornstarch
1 onion, diced
1/3 c. creamy peanut butter
3 c. cooked vermicelli pasta

Combine turkey, green pepper, one cup broth, soy sauce, garlic and red pepper flakes in a slow cooker. Cover and cook on low setting for 3 to 4 hours, until juices run clear. Mix cornstarch with remaining broth until smooth; stir into slow cooker. Add onion and peanut butter; mix well. Turn slow cooker to high setting; cover and cook for an additional 30 minutes. Serve over cooked vermicelli.

Nutrition Per Serving: 336 calories, 9g total fat, 2g sat fat, 45mg cholesterol, 630mg sodium, 29g carbohydrate, 3g fiber, 37g protein

Debby Conaway, Rome, GA

Debby's Chicken Lasagna

This delicious recipe takes just four hours...pretty fast for a slow-cooker recipe. It's great on hectic days and you are in a pinch for time. Feel free to double the recipe if your slow cooker is large enough.

Makes 8 servings

3 6-oz. boneless, skinless chicken
   breasts, cooked and shredded
26-oz. jar spaghetti sauce
9-oz. pkg. lasagna noodles, uncooked
   and divided
1 c. low-fat ricotta cheese, divided
1 c. shredded part-skim mozzarella
   cheese, divided
1 c. shredded reduced-fat Cheddar
   cheese

In a bowl, mix chicken with sauce. Layer in an oval slow cooker as follows: 1/3 of chicken mixture, 1/3 of uncooked noodles, 1/3 of ricotta cheese and 1/3 of mozzarella cheese. Break noodles to fit as they are needed. Repeat layering twice; top with Cheddar cheese. Cover and cook on high setting for 3 hours. Turn setting to low; continue cooking for one hour, or until bubbly and noodles are tender.

Nutrition Per Serving: 356 calories, 11g total fat, 5g sat fat, 77mg cholesterol, 705mg sodium, 32g carbohydrate, 3g fiber, 31g protein

Liz Plotnick-Snay, Gooseberry Patch

Slow-Cooker Tagine Chicken

My husband and I love to try all different types of food...Thai, Indian, Lebanese, you name it. We both really enjoyed this tasty dish. To make it ahead, combine all the ingredients except broth and couscous and refrigerate overnight or freeze until ready to use. If frozen, thaw before cooking in slow cooker.

Makes 6 servings

2 lbs. boneless, skinless chicken
   breasts, cubed
1 T. ground coriander
1 T. paprika
1 T. ground cumin
1 t. turmeric
1/8 t. cinnamon
1 c. onion, diced
3/4 c. water
3/4 c. raisins
3/4 c. prunes
14-oz. can chicken broth
2 c. cooked couscous

In a bowl, toss chicken with spices. Combine chicken, onion, water, raisins, prunes and broth into a slow cooker. Cover and cook on low setting for 8 to 9 hours. Serve over couscous.

Nutrition Per Serving: 368 calories, 4g total fat, 1g sat fat, 110mg cholesterol, 345mg sodium, 45g carbohydrate, 4g fiber, 38g protein

★ LOW-CAL ADD-ON ★ **Top each serving with 2 tablespoons non-fat plain Greek yogurt for an additional 20 calories per serving.**

Dawn Dhooghe, Concord, NC

Bayou Chicken

The slow cooker always seems to be going at our house. This is one of my husband's favorite meals...and it's so easy to put together!

Makes 6 servings

4 6-oz. boneless, skinless chicken breasts, cubed
14-1/2 oz. can low-sodium chicken broth
14-1/2 oz. can diced tomatoes
10-3/4 oz. can tomato soup
1/2 lb. smoked turkey sausage, sliced
1/2 c. cooked lean ham, diced
1 onion, chopped
2 t. Cajun seasoning
hot pepper sauce to taste
3 c. cooked brown rice

Combine all ingredients except rice in a slow cooker; stir. Cover and cook on low setting for 7 to 8 hours. Serve chicken mixture over hot cooked rice.

Nutrition Per Serving: 396 calories, 9g total fat, 2g sat fat, 119mg cholesterol, 951mg sodium, 37g carbohydrate, 3g fiber, 39g protein

★ LOW-CAL ADD-ON ★ Sprinkle with any chopped fresh herb you have on hand like parsley, rosemary or thyme for a zero-calorie garnish.

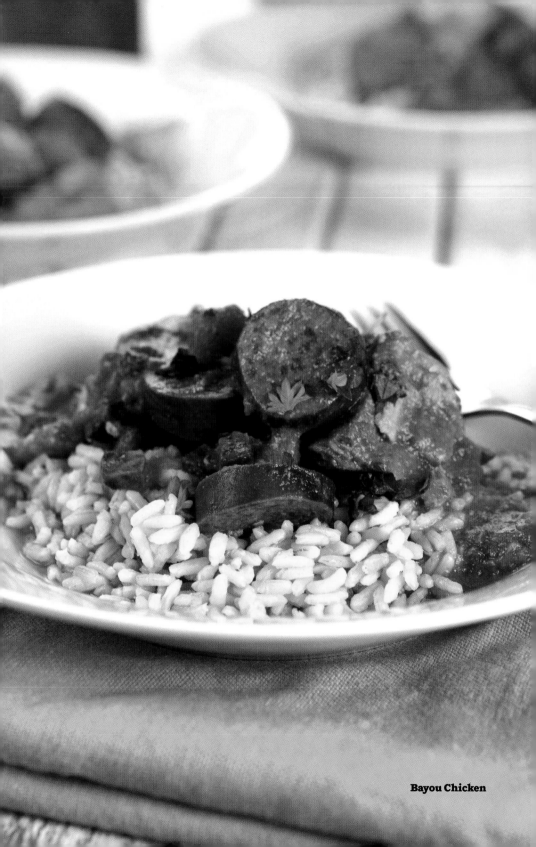

Bayou Chicken

Mindy Humphrey, Evansville, IN

Mexican Dump Chicken

Toss this simple recipe into the slow cooker first thing in the morning. Hardly any prep is required! Leftovers freeze well too.

Makes 6 servings

2 6-oz. boneless, skinless chicken breasts
15-oz. can corn, drained
15-oz. can black beans, drained and rinsed
8-oz. jar salsa
1 onion, coarsely chopped
8-oz. pkg. 1/3-less-fat cream cheese, cubed
6-oz. pkg. multi-grain tortilla chips

Place chicken breasts in a slow cooker. Top with corn, beans, salsa and onion. Cover and cook on low setting for 6 to 8 hours, until chicken is tender. About 30 minutes before serving, shred chicken in slow cooker. Add cream cheese; stir to combine. Cover and cook on low setting for 30 minutes, or until cream cheese has melted. Serve chicken mixture with tortilla chips.

Nutrition Per Serving: 381 calories, 19g total fat, 6g sat fat, 69mg cholesterol, 802mg sodium, 33g carbohydrate, 6g fiber, 22g protein

Barbara Hightower, Broomfield, CO

Healthy Crock Burritos

My daughter Gigi gave me this easy recipe for chicken burritos after she served them to us for family dinner at her house. Great for filling up the slow cooker and coming home to a hot meal...they're low-calorie and really delicious.

Makes 6 servings

4 6-oz. boneless, skinless chicken
   breasts
15-oz. can black beans, drained and
   rinsed
15-1/4 oz. can corn, rinsed and
   drained
7-oz. can red enchilada sauce
7-oz. can green enchilada sauce
6 burrito-size whole-wheat flour
   tortillas
Garnish: chopped onions, shredded
   lettuce, sour cream, shredded
   Cheddar cheese

Arrange chicken breasts in a slow cooker. Layer beans, corn and sauces over chicken. Cover and cook on low setting for 6 to 8 hours. Remove chicken to a plate; shred with a fork. Return chicken to slow cooker and stir to mix. To serve, spoon chicken mixture into tortillas; add desired toppings and roll up.

Nutrition Per Serving: 343 calories, 7g total fat, 2g sat fat, 83mg cholesterol, 920mg sodium, 36g carbohydrate, 7g fiber, 22g protein

Tricia Roberson, Indian Head, MD

Frank's Chicken

The mouthwatering gravy is tasty over rice.

Makes 6 servings

4 potatoes, peeled and quartered
1 carrot, peeled and chopped
1 onion, diced
1 stalk celery, chopped
2 lbs. skinless chicken legs and
   thighs
1/2 c. low-sodium chicken broth
1/4 c. white wine or low-sodium
   chicken broth
1/2 T. paprika
2 t. garlic powder
1/2 t. dried rosemary
1/2 t. dried basil
Optional: 2 to 3 T. cornstarch

Place vegetables in a slow cooker; arrange chicken on top. Pour chicken broth and wine or additional broth over all; sprinkle with seasonings. Cover and cook on low setting for 8 hours, or on high setting for 5 hours. Remove chicken and vegetables to a serving platter. If gravy is desired, stir cornstarch into juices in slow cooker. Cook until thickened.

Nutrition Per Serving: 304 calories, 7g total fat, 2g sat fat, 140mg cholesterol, 174mg sodium, 26g carbohydrate, 3g fiber, 33g protein

★ LOW-CAL ADD-ON ★ Spoon each serving over 1/2 cup of piping-hot cooked brown rice for an extra 125 calories.

Debi Piper, Vicksburg, MI

Chicken Stew Over Biscuits

This creamy chicken dish is a cross between a stew and a hearty gravy that's served over buttermilk biscuits.

Makes 8 servings

2 c. water
1 to 2 t. chicken bouillon granules
3/4 c. white wine or chicken broth
2 0.87-oz. pkgs. chicken gravy mix
2 cloves garlic, minced
1 T. fresh parsley, minced
1/2 t. pepper
1 onion, cut into 8 wedges
5 carrots, peeled and cut into 1-inch pieces
2 lbs. skinless, boneless chicken breasts, cut into bite-size pieces
3 T. all-purpose flour
1/3 c. cold water
16.3-oz. tube refrigerated large buttermilk biscuits, baked

Combine first 7 ingredients in a slow cooker; mix until blended. Add onion, carrots and chicken; cover and cook on low setting for 7 to 8 hours. In a bowl, stir together flour and cold water until smooth; gradually stir into slow cooker. Increase setting to high; cover and cook for one hour. Place biscuits in soup bowls; top with stew.

Nutrition Per Serving: 376 calories, 11g total fat, 4g sat fat, 83mg cholesterol, 997mg sodium, 33g carbohydrate, 2g fiber, 31g protein

★ SAVVY SWAP ★ Sub 2 cups of chicken broth for the 2 cups of water and the chicken bouillon granules.

Anne Alesauskas, Minocqua, WI

Cashew Chicken

This is one of the simplest recipes in my recipe box and I think you'll love it! We just love Chinese foods... unfortunately, our options aren't great for take-out, so I make my own whenever possible. Using the slow cooker is an added bonus on those days when you're running like mad.

Makes 4 servings

1/4 c. all-purpose flour
1/8 t. pepper
1 lb. boneless, skinless chicken
    breasts, cubed
1 T. canola oil
1/4 c. low-sodium soy sauce
2 T. rice wine vinegar
2 T. catsup
1 T. brown sugar, packed
1 clove garlic, minced
1/2 t. fresh ginger, peeled and grated
red pepper flakes to taste
2 c. cooked brown rice
1/4 c. cashews

Combine flour and pepper in a plastic zipping bag. Add chicken pieces to bag; toss to coat. Remove chicken from bag and shake to remove excess flour mixture. Heat oil in a large skillet over medium-high heat. Cook chicken for about 5 minutes, until golden on all sides but not cooked through. Transfer chicken to a slow cooker; set aside. In a small bowl, combine remaining ingredients except rice and cashews. Pour mixture over chicken, stirring slightly. Cover and cook on low setting for 3 to 4 hours, or on high setting for one to 2 hours, until chicken juices run clear. To serve, spoon chicken mixture over cooked rice; top with cashews.

Nutrition Per Serving: 398 calories, 11g total fat, 2g sat fat, 83mg cholesterol, 876mg sodium, 42g carbohydrate, 2g fiber, 31g protein

★ LOW-CAL ADD-ON ★ Serve with lime wedges and chopped fresh cilantro for a burst of bright, fresh flavor.

Nola Coons, Gooseberry Patch

Rosemary-Garlic Tenderloins

If the aroma isn't enough to pull you in, one bite and you'll find these turkey tenderloins amazingly juicy and full of flavor.

Makes 6 servings

1-1/4 c. white wine or low-sodium chicken broth
1 onion, chopped
2 cloves garlic, minced
2 bay leaves
2 t. dried rosemary
1/2 t. pepper
2 lbs. boneless, skinless turkey breast tenderloins
3 T. cornstarch
1/2 c. half-and-half or 2% reduced-fat milk
1/2 t. salt

Combine wine or broth, onion, garlic and bay leaves in a slow cooker. Mix together rosemary and pepper; rub over turkey. Place in a slow cooker. Cover and cook on low setting for 7 to 8 hours, or until a meat thermometer inserted in thickest part of turkey reads 170 degrees. Remove turkey and keep warm. Strain cooking juices into a saucepan. Combine cornstarch, half-and-half or milk and salt until smooth; gradually add to saucepan. Bring to a boil over medium heat; cook and stir for 2 minutes, until thickened. Remove and discard bay leaves. Slice turkey; serve with sauce.

Nutrition Per Serving: 248 calories, 4g total fat, 1g sat fat, 67mg cholesterol, 294mg sodium, 8g carbohydrate, 1g fiber, 38g protein

Carrie O'Shea, Marina Del Rey, CA

Thai Chicken & Rice

Makes 6 servings

4 6-oz. boneless, skinless chicken
   breasts or thighs, cut into strips
1 red pepper, sliced
1 onion, coarsely chopped
1/2 c. low-sodium chicken broth
5 T. low-sodium soy sauce, divided
3 cloves garlic, minced
1 T. ground cumin
1/2 t. salt
1/2 t. pepper
2 T. cornstarch
1/2 c. creamy peanut butter
3 T. lime juice
3 c. cooked brown rice
Garnish: chopped fresh cilantro,
   chopped green onions, chopped
   peanuts

Arrange chicken, red pepper and onion in a slow cooker; set aside. In a bowl, combine broth and 4 tablespoons soy sauce; drizzle over chicken mixture. Add garlic and seasonings to slow cooker; stir to mix. Cover and cook on low setting for 4-1/2 to 5 hours, until chicken is no longer pink in the center. Remove 1/2 cup liquid from slow cooker; mix with cornstarch, peanut butter, lime juice and remaining soy sauce in a bowl. Stir mixture back into slow cooker; increase heat to high setting. Cover and cook for 30 minutes. Spoon over cooked rice to serve; garnish as desired.

Nutrition Per Serving: 391 calories, 14g total fat, 3g sat fat, 62mg cholesterol, 817mg sodium, 38g carbohydrate, 4g fiber, 28g protein

★ LOW-CAL ADD-ON ★ **Peanuts add a nice crunch to this dish. Sprinkle one tablespoon over each serving for an extra 50 calories.**

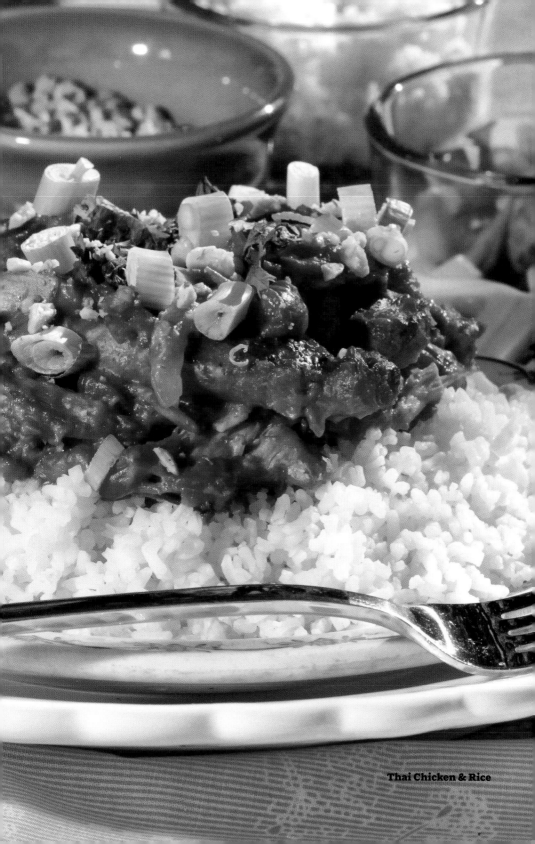

Thai Chicken & Rice

Melanie Lowe, Dover DE

Buffalo Chicken Potato Skins

These treats are my son's favorite. He loves buffalo chicken everything, and since these are so easy to make, I have no problem making them for him when he asks...which is quite often!

Makes 6 servings

1 lb. boneless, skinless chicken
   breasts
1/2 onion, chopped
1 clove garlic, minced
1 stalk celery, chopped
14-1/2 oz. can low-sodium chicken
   broth
1/3 c. cayenne hot pepper sauce
6 8-oz. baking potatoes, baked
1/2 t. salt
1/2 t. pepper
3/4 c. reduced-fat shredded Cheddar
   cheese
Garnish: yogurt blue cheese salad
   dressing

Combine chicken, onion, garlic, celery and broth in a slow cooker. Cover and cook on high setting for 4 hours, or until chicken is no longer pink in the center. Remove and shred chicken, reserving 1/2 cup juices from slow cooker, discarding the rest. Combine shredded chicken, reserved juices and hot sauce in slow cooker. Cover and cook on high setting for 30 minutes. Meanwhile, slice baked potatoes in half lengthwise; scoop out pulp and save for another recipe. Place potato skins on a lightly greased baking sheet. Lightly spray skins with non-stick vegetable spray; sprinkle with salt and pepper. Bake at

450 degrees for 10 minutes, or until lightly golden. Evenly divide chicken mixture and Cheddar cheese among potato skins. Bake again for about 5 minutes, until cheese is melted. Drizzle potatoes with dressing before serving.

Nutrition Per Serving: 301 calories, 5g fat, 2g sat fat, 65mg cholesterol, 721mg sodium, 38g carbohydrate, 4g fiber, 26g protein

Kristi Duis, Maple Plain, NY

Fiesta Chicken Pronto

We like to serve this spicy chicken in burritos...mini tacos are fun for parties too!

Makes 8 servings

8 6-oz. boneless, skinless chicken
   breasts
16-oz. can black beans, drained and
   rinsed
10-3/4 oz. can cream of chicken soup
2 T. taco seasoning mix
1/4 c. salsa
16 corn taco shells
Garnish: diced tomatoes, sliced
   jalapeño peppers, sliced olives

Arrange chicken in a slow cooker. Combine remaining ingredients except taco shells and garnish; pour over chicken. Cover and cook on high setting for 3 hours. Remove chicken; shred and stir back into slow cooker. Spoon into taco shells; garnish as desired.

Nutrition Per Serving: 372 calories, 12g total fat, 4g sat fat, 138mg cholesterol, 627mg sodium, 21g carbohydrate, 4g fiber, 42g protein

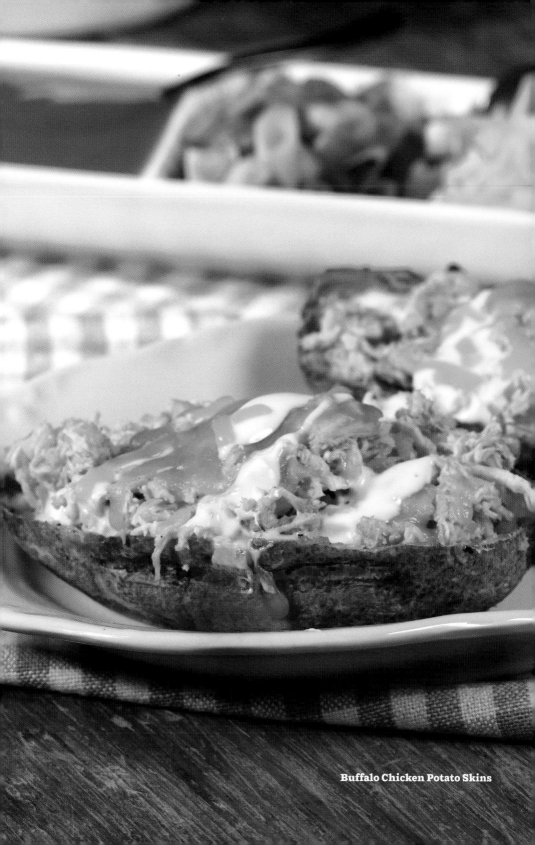

Buffalo Chicken Potato Skins

Wendy Lee Paffenroth, Pine Island, NY

Divine Chicken

I created this slow-cooker recipe one morning with the foods I had on hand, and my family loved it! Substitute whole-grain pasta for the rice, if desired.

Makes 6 servings

3 6-oz. boneless, skinless chicken breasts, cut in half
2 10-3/4 oz. cans cream of chicken soup
1-1/4 c. 1% low-fat milk
3 c. frozen carrots
1-1/2 c. frozen broccoli flowerets
1-1/2 oz. pkg. onion soup mix
3 c. cooked brown rice

Mix together all ingredients except rice or pasta in a slow cooker. Cover and cook on low setting for 6 to 8 hours. Using a slotted spoon, arrange chicken and vegetables on cooked rice. Top with sauce from slow cooker.

Nutrition Per Serving: 376 calories, 11g total fat, 2g sat fat, 62mg cholesterol, 1197mg sodium, 44g carbohydrate, 5g fiber, 25g protein

★ SAVVY SWAP ★ Frozen green beans make a good stand-in for the frozen broccoli.

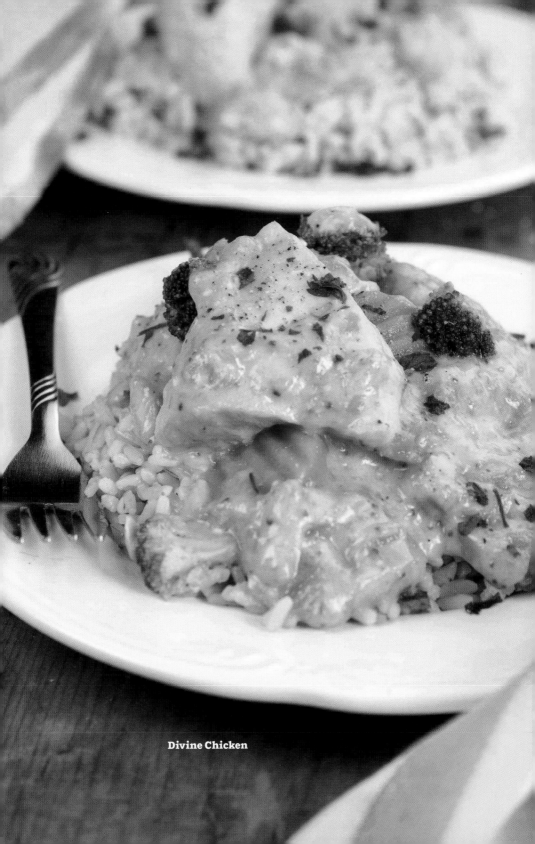

Divine Chicken

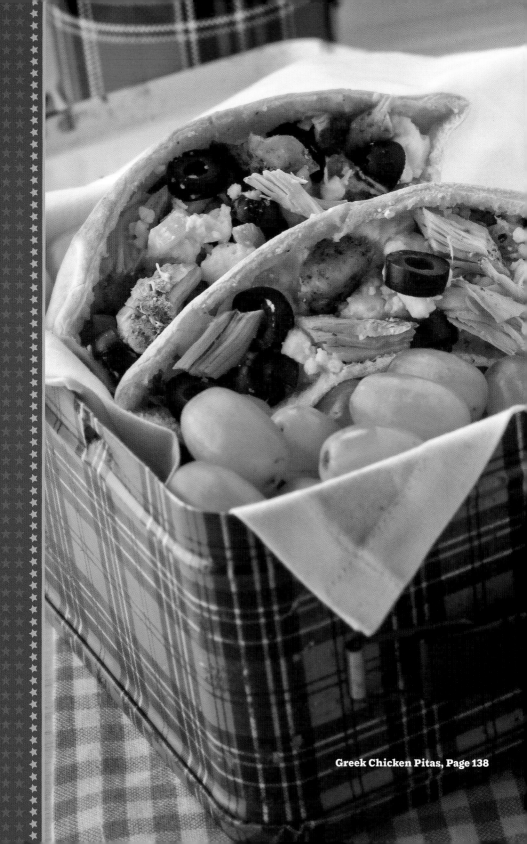

Greek Chicken Pitas, Page 138

CHAPTER FIVE

Sandwiches

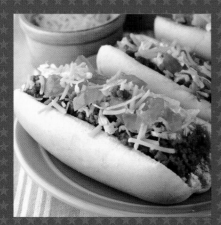

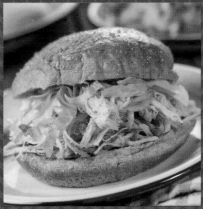

Tex-Mex Taco Joes, Page 130

Shredded Chicken Sandwiches, Page 142

Virginia Watson, Scranton, PA

Meatball Hoagies

Hoagies, submarines, grinders, po' boys...whatever you call 'em, just call us for dinner!

Makes 8 servings

1 lb. lean ground beef
1/2 c. Italian-flavored dry bread
   crumbs
1 egg, beaten
2 T. onion, minced
1 T. grated Parmesan cheese
1 t. salt
1 t. Worcestershire sauce
32-oz. jar pasta sauce
8 2-1/2-oz. hoagie rolls, split
Garnish: sliced mozzarella cheese

In a large bowl, combine beef, bread crumbs, egg, onion, Parmesan cheese, salt and Worcestershire sauce. Using your hands, mix just until combined. Form into one-inch meatballs. Cook meatballs in a large skillet, turning occasionally, until browned on all sides. Remove meatballs to a slow cooker; top with pasta sauce. Cover and cook on low setting for about 2 hours, stirring after one hour. To serve, spoon several meatballs into each bun; top with a spoonful of sauce and a slice of cheese.

Nutrition Per Serving: 383 calories, 11g total fat, 4g sat fat, 59mg cholesterol, 779mg sodium, 49g carbohydrate, 4g fiber, 23g protein

★ LOW-CAL ADD-ON ★ **If you want to add cheese to this sandwich, an 0.8-ounce slice will add 60 calories.**

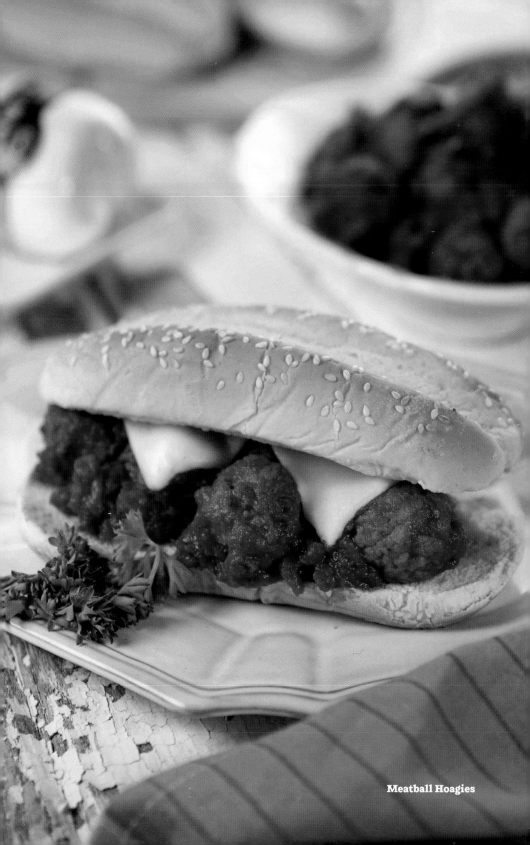

Meatball Hoagies

Kathy White, Cato, NY

Easy French Dip Sandwiches

My husband is the pastor of our church and our family of ten regularly hosts meals with the congregation. These hearty sandwiches feed a crowd!

Makes 20 servings

4 lbs. stew beef cubes
2 onions, halved
4 cloves garlic
2-1/2 c. low-sodium beef broth
4 t. beef bouillon granules
20 2-oz. whole-wheat sandwich
   buns, split

Combine all ingredients except buns in a slow cooker. Cover and cook on low setting for 8 to 10 hours. Discard onions and garlic. Remove beef to a bowl and shred; spoon onto buns. Serve with beef juices from cooker for dipping.

Nutrition Per Serving: 267 calories, 6g total fat, 2g sat fat, 61mg cholesterol, 474mg sodium, 26g carbohydrate, 4g fiber, 20g protein

---

★ SKINNY SECRET ★ Stew beef cubes are a leaner cut of meat, which makes it a great choice when watching calories. Cooking it low and slow for a long time is the key to making this tougher cut fork-tender.

Ann Mathis, Biscoe, AR

Philly Cheesesteaks

We have made these sandwiches on a large scale and sold them at concession stands. They would sell out in an hour or less. The more thinly sliced the beef is, the less cooking time required.

Makes 8 servings

2-lb. beef round steak, thinly sliced
1/2 t. pepper
1/2 t. garlic powder
1 onion, sliced
1 green pepper, sliced
4 c. low-sodium beef broth
8 1-3/4 oz. French rolls, sliced
8 3/4-oz. slices provolone or
   American cheese, cut in half

Rub beef slices with pepper and garlic powder. Place in a slow cooker; add onion, green pepper and beef broth. Stir to mix. Cover and cook on low setting for 5 to 7 hours, until beef is tender. At serving time, toast rolls on a baking sheet in a 350-degree oven. To serve, lay a cheese half-slice on both sides of each roll. Top cheese with beef mixture, using tongs to remove beef mixture with onion and pepper onto rolls, letting juices drip back into slow cooker. Return sandwiches to oven for a few minutes, until cheese is melted.

Nutrition Per Serving: 381 calories, 14g total fat, 6g sat fat, 91mg cholesterol, 540mg sodium, 28g carbohydrate, 2g fiber, 35g protein

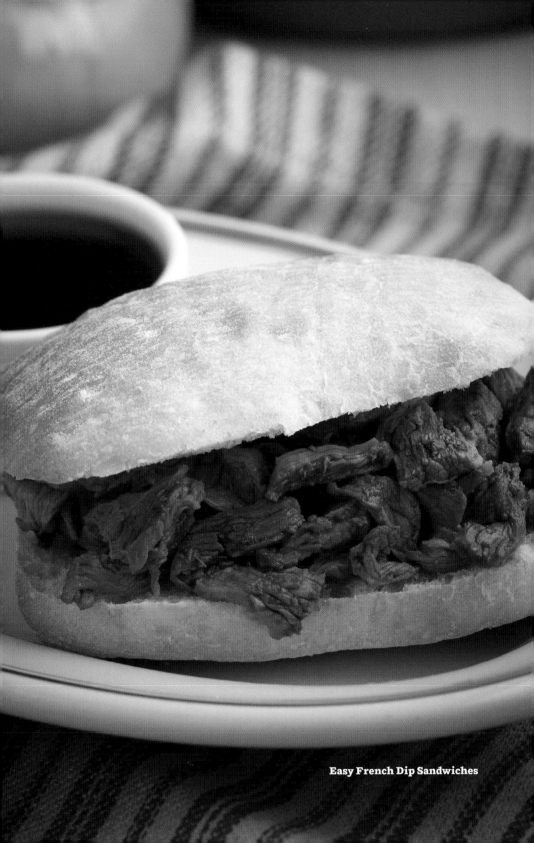

Easy French Dip Sandwiches

Sherry Cress, Salem, IN

Tex-Mex Taco Joes

A super-simple meal that's full of flavor. Try garnishing with a little peach or pineapple salsa...really good!

Makes 25 servings

3 lbs. lean ground beef, browned and
    drained
16-oz. can refried beans
10-oz can enchilada sauce
1-1/4 oz. pkg. taco seasoning mix
16-oz. jar salsa
25 2-oz. whole-wheat hot dog buns,
    split
Garnish: shredded Cheddar cheese,
    shredded lettuce, chopped
    tomatoes, sour cream

Place beef in a slow cooker. Stir in beans, enchilada sauce, seasoning mix and salsa. Cover and cook on low setting for 4 to 6 hours. To serve, fill each bun with 1/3 cup beef mixture; garnish as desired.

Nutrition Per Serving: 250 calories, 6g total fat, 2g sat fat, 34mg cholesterol, 739mg sodium, 28g carbohydrate, 7g fiber, 20g protein

★ LOW-CAL ADD-ON ★ Pile on the chopped tomatoes and shredded lettuce as each of these items will add minimal calories. But watch the sour cream and cheese...one tablespoon of both will add 60 more calories to each serving.

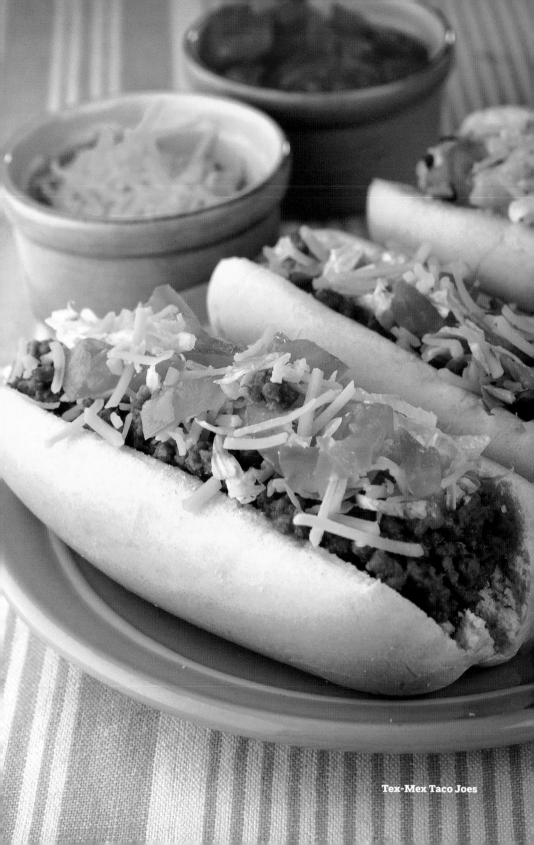

Tex-Mex Taco Joes

Carolyn Deckard, Bedford, IN

Jim's Sloppy Joes

Knowing this is my favorite sandwich, my husband would fix these easy Sloppy Joes when we were working on different shifts.

Makes 12 servings

3 lbs. lean ground beef
1 onion, finely chopped
1 T. garlic, minced
1-1/2 c. catsup
1/4 c. brown sugar, packed
3-1/2 T. mustard
3 T. Worcestershire sauce
1 T. chili powder
2 stalks celery, chopped
12 2-oz. whole-wheat sandwich buns, split
Optional: pickles or coleslaw

In a large skillet over medium heat, brown beef with onion and garlic; drain. Meanwhile, spray a 5-quart slow cooker with non-stick vegetable spray. Add remaining ingredients except buns to slow cooker; mix well. Stir in beef mixture. Cover and cook on low setting for 6 to 7 hours. To serve, spoon beef mixture onto buns. Top with pickles or a spoonful of coleslaw, if desired.

Nutrition Per Serving: 376 calories, 10g total fat, 4g sat fat, 72mg cholesterol, 624mg sodium, 40g carbohydrate, 4g fiber, 24g protein

Virginia Watson, Scranton, PA

Teriyaki Steak Subs

We really enjoy these sandwiches at all our winter tailgating parties. They're great for an easy dinner too.

Makes 10 servings

1/2 c. onion, chopped
1/2 c. low-sodium soy sauce
1/4 c. red wine or low-sodium beef broth
1 T. fresh ginger, peeled and grated
1 T. sugar
3 lbs. beef round steak, cut crosswise into thirds
10 2-1/2 oz. sub buns, split
Garnish: thinly sliced onion

In a bowl, combine all ingredients except buns and garnish. Layer beef pieces in a slow cooker, spoon some of the onion mixture over each piece. Cover and cook on low setting for 6 to 7 hours, until beef is tender. Remove beef to a platter, reserving cooking liquid in slow cooker. Let beef stand several minutes before thinly slicing. To serve, place sliced beef on buns; top with sliced onion and some of the reserved cooking liquid.

Nutrition Per Serving: 383 calories, 12g total fat, 4g sat fat, 63mg cholesterol, 844mg sodium, 37g carbohydrate, 2g fiber, 28g protein

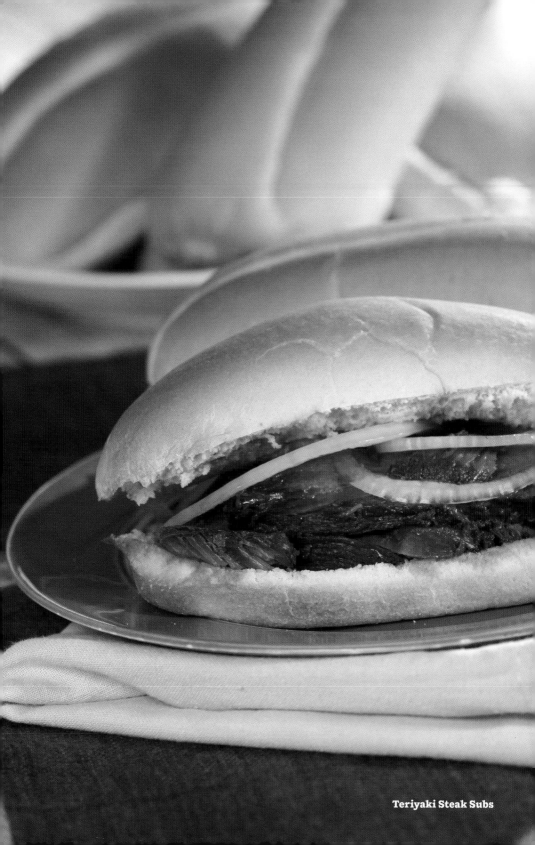

Teriyaki Steak Subs

Melanie Foster, North Wilkesboro, NC

Pulled Pork Barbecue

This is a budget-friendly, family-pleasing main dish that is requested often in my home.

Makes 16 servings

1-3/4 c. low-sodium beef broth
1/2 c. regular or non-alcoholic beer
4-lb. Boston butt pork roast
18-oz. bottle smoke-flavored barbecue sauce
16 2-oz. whole-wheat sandwich buns, split

Pour broth and beer into a large slow cooker; add roast. Cover and cook on high setting for 4 hours, or on low setting for 8 hours, until roast is very tender. Remove roast from slow cooker. Shred roast with 2 forks and transfer to a roasting pan. Stir in barbecue sauce. Bake, uncovered, at 350 degrees for 30 minutes. Fill buns with pulled pork to make sandwiches.

Nutrition Per Serving: 239 calories, 10g total fat, 4g sat fat, 268mg cholesterol, 542mg sodium, 22g carbohydrate, 2g fiber, 15g protein

★ LOW-CAL ADD-ON ★ **Pair each sandwich with 1/4 cup slaw and 1/4 cup baked beans for an additional 175 calories.**

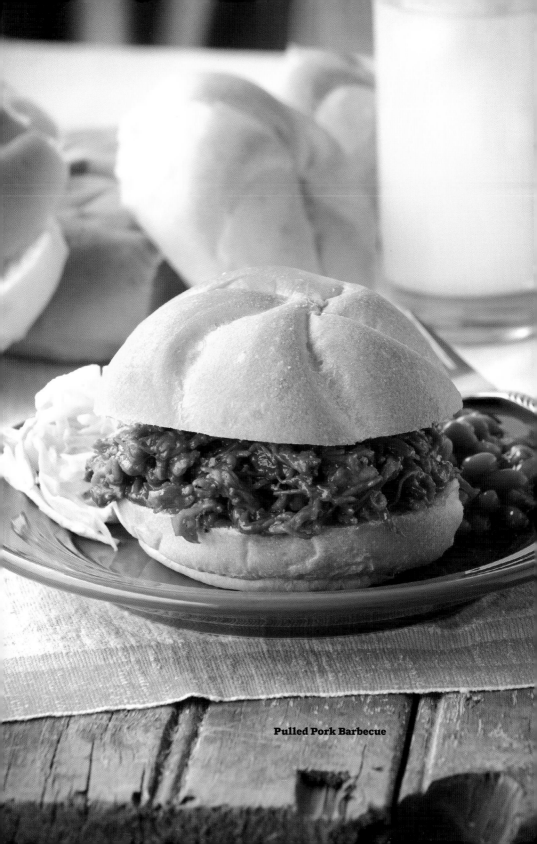

Pulled Pork Barbecue

Marie Matter, Dallas, TX

Simple Spiced Pulled Pork

This is my go-to recipe for pulled pork. It's delicious in everything like sandwiches, enchiladas, tacos...you name it! The roast's juices will slowly release as it cooks, so you don't even need to add any liquid to your slow cooker. So easy!

Makes 8 servings

2-lb. boneless pork shoulder roast
3 T. chili powder
1 T. smoked paprika
1 T. kosher salt
2 t. ground cumin
1 t. dried oregano
1 t. onion powder
1 t. garlic powder
1/2 t. cayenne pepper
1/4 t. cinnamon
1 T. light brown sugar, packed
2 t. canola oil
8 2-oz. whole-wheat sandwich buns, split

Pat roast dry with paper towels; set aside. Combine spices and brown sugar in a small bowl; mix well. Rub spice mix all over roast; set aside any remaining spice mix. Heat oil in a large skillet over medium-high heat. Brown roast on all sides for one to 2 minutes per side. Transfer roast to a slow cooker; sprinkle with remaining spice mix. Cover and cook on low setting for 6 to 10 hours, to desired tenderness. Remove roast to a plate; shred with 2 forks or cut into small pieces. Serve pork in buns.

Nutrition Per Serving: 349 calories, 14g total fat, 5g sat fat, 67mg cholesterol, 1001mg sodium, 26g carbohydrate, 3g fiber, 19g protein

Bethi Hendrickson, Danville, PA

Auntie B's BBQ Roast Sandwiches

This recipe is a favorite for quick suppers or large groups. You can use a pork roast instead of beef in this recipe too...both are fantastic. Serve on hearty rolls and you have a winner.

Makes 12 servings

4-lb. lean beef chuck roast, fat trimmed
1 c. tomato juice
1/4 c. Worcestershire sauce
1 T. white vinegar
1 t. dry mustard
1 t. chili powder
1/4 t. garlic powder
12 1-3/4 oz. hearty whole-grain rolls, split

Spray a slow cooker with non-stick vegetable spray; add roast and set aside. In a small bowl, combine remaining ingredients except rolls. Stir until mixed well; pour over roast. Cover and cook on low setting for 8 to 10 hours, or on high setting for 5 to 6 hours, until roast is very tender. Shred roast with 2 forks. Serve beef on rolls, drizzled with a little of the sauce from slow cooker.

Nutrition Per Serving: 285 calories, 7g total fat, 2g sat fat, 88mg cholesterol, 364mg sodium, 19g carbohydrate, 1g fiber, 34g protein

★ LOW-CAL ADD-ON ★ **For a crunchy and salty side, partner sandwiches with one ounce baked potato chips for an extra 120 calories per serving.**

Peggy Pelfrey, Ashland City, TN

Greek Chicken Pitas

For a real treat, top these pitas with some crumbled feta cheese and sliced black olives.

Makes 8 servings

1 onion, diced
3 cloves garlic, minced
1 lb. boneless, skinless chicken
   breasts, cut into strips
1 t. lemon pepper seasoning
1/2 t. dried oregano
1/4 c. low-fat plain yogurt
1/4 c. reduced-fat sour cream
1/2 c. cucumber, peeled and diced
4 3-oz. rounds wheat pita bread,
   halved and split

Place onion and garlic in a slow cooker; set aside. Sprinkle chicken with seasonings; add to slow cooker. Cover and cook on high setting for 5 to 6 hours. Meanwhile, stir together yogurt, sour cream and cucumber in a small bowl; chill. Fill pita halves with chicken mixture and drizzle with yogurt sauce.

Nutrition Per Serving: 210 calories, 4g total fat, 1g sat fat, 45mg cholesterol, 248mg sodium, 26g carbohydrate, 3g fiber, 19g protein

★ LOW-CAL ADD-ON ★ **Round out your meal with one cup of sweet and juicy seedless grapes for an additional 100 calories.**

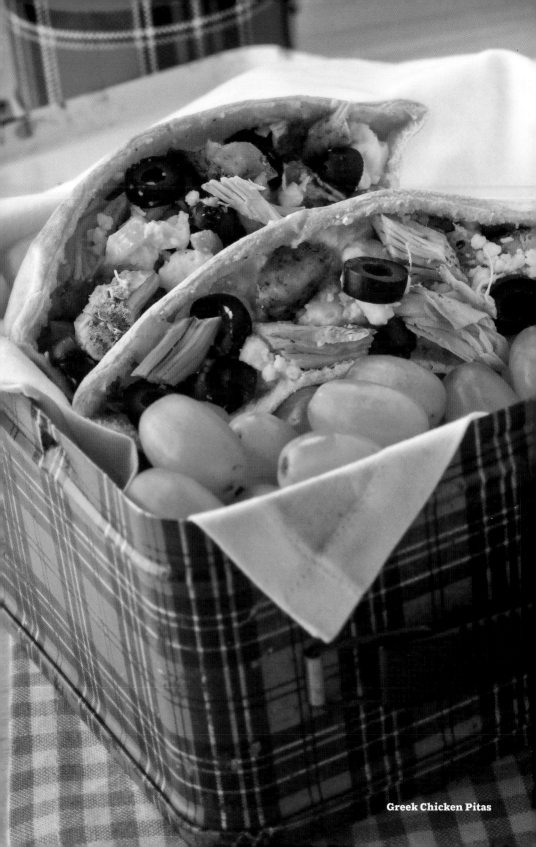

Greek Chicken Pitas

DonnaMarie Ebhardt, Davenport, FL

Spicy Buffalo Chicken Sloppy Joes

I experimented with a buffalo chicken recipe and tweaked it to make Sloppy Joes...yum!

Makes 8 servings

1-1/2 T. extra-virgin olive oil
2 lbs. ground or shredded chicken breast
1 c. green, red and/or yellow peppers, chopped
1 onion, chopped
1 T. garlic, minced
1/2 c. tomato sauce
1/4 c. low-sodium chicken broth
1/4 c. thick-style hot buffalo wing sauce
2 T. brown sugar, packed
2 T. dry mustard
1-1/2 t. chili powder
8-oz. pkg. shredded reduced-fat Mexican-style cheese
8 2-oz. whole-wheat sandwich buns, split
Garnish: lettuce leaves, sliced tomatoes, crumbled blue cheese

Heat olive oil in a large skillet over medium-high heat; stir in chicken. Cook until crumbly, golden and no longer pink. Remove chicken to a 5-quart slow cooker. Stir in remaining ingredients except buns and garnish. Cover and cook on low setting for 4 to 5 hours. During the last 30 minutes, turn slow cooker to high setting; cook and stir mixture to desired thickness. Serve chicken mixture on buns, garnished with lettuce, tomato and a sprinkle of blue cheese. May omit buns; serve on lettuce-lined plates, garnished as desired.

Nutrition Per Serving: 397 calories, 12g total fat, 4g sat fat, 81mg cholesterol, 555mg sodium, 32g carbohydrate, 4g fiber, 35g protein

Tina Elyea, Greenwood, NE

Carolyn's Italian Beef

This is from my mother-in-law Carolyn. She likes to tell the story about the time she had a group of ladies over lunch and served them the "juice" from the recipe as a soup. The ladies raved about it!

Makes 12 servings

4-lb. beef chuck roast, fat trimmed
1 T. onion, minced
2 t. garlic powder
2 t. dried oregano
2 t. dried rosemary
1 t. caraway seed
1 t. celery seed
1 t. salt
1/4 t. cayenne pepper
12 1-3/4 oz. hearty whole-grain rolls, split

Place roast in a large slow cooker; set aside. In a small bowl, combine onion and seasonings; rub mixture over roast. Add enough water to cover roast. Cover and cook on low setting for about 10 hours. Shred roast with 2 forks, discarding any fat. Serve beef mixture spooned into rolls.

Nutrition Per Serving: 297 calories, 7g total fat, 2g sat fat, 88mg cholesterol, 475mg sodium, 21g carbohydrate, 1g fiber, 34g protein

Vickie, Gooseberry Patch

Shredded Chicken Sandwiches

Tender chicken piled high on a soft bun...just like the sandwiches at old-fashioned church socials.

Makes 8 servings

1/4 c. olive oil

4 6-oz. boneless, skinless chicken breasts

1 onion, chopped

10-3/4 oz. can cream of mushroom soup

1 c. low-sodium chicken broth

1/2 c. sherry or low-sodium chicken broth

2 t. low-sodium soy sauce

2 t. Worcestershire sauce

1/2 t. salt

1/2 t. pepper

8 2-oz. whole-wheat sandwich buns, split

Optional: pickle slices, lettuce leaves

Heat oil in a skillet over medium-high heat. Add chicken. Cook for 5 minutes on each side, until golden. Transfer chicken to a slow cooker; set aside. Add onion to drippings in skillet. Sauté until golden; drain. Add soup, broth, sherry or broth, sauces and seasonings to skillet. Stir mixture well and spoon over chicken in slow cooker. Cover and cook on low setting for 7 to 8 hours. Shred chicken with a fork; spoon onto buns. Garnish with pickles and lettuce, if desired.

Nutrition Per Serving: 369 calories, 13g total fat, 2g sat fat, 63mg cholesterol, 829mg sodium, 30g carbohydrate, 4g fiber, 20g protein

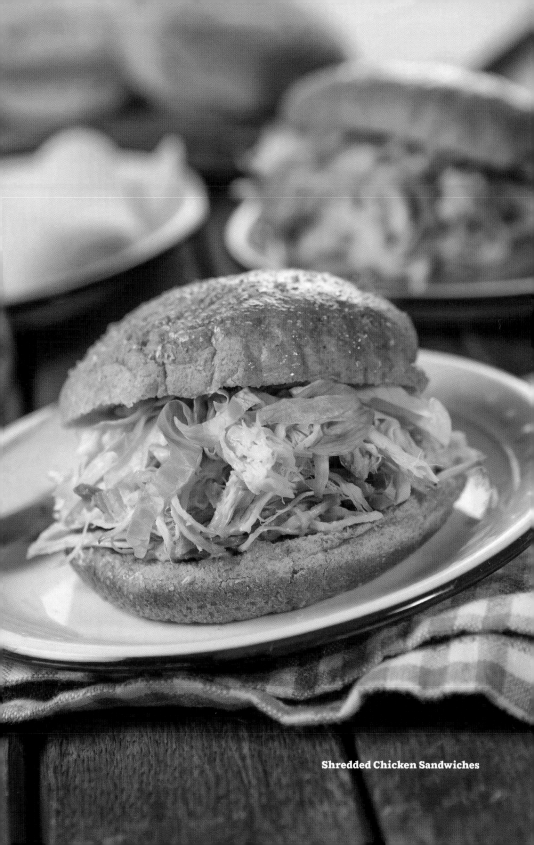

Shredded Chicken Sandwiches

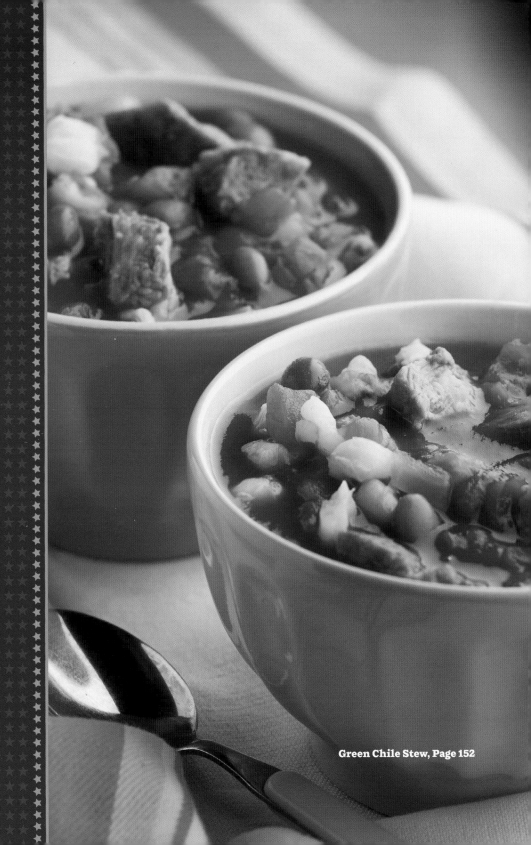

Green Chile Stew, Page 152

CHAPTER SIX

Soups & Stews

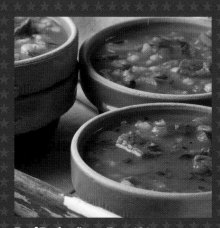

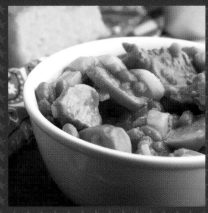

Beef Barley Soup, Page 164

Chuck Wagon Stew, Page 160

Barbara Cebula, Chicopee, MA

Barb's Corn Chowder

I make this on a fall day when I want something hot, creamy and delicious for my family. They love it! When sweet corn isn't in season, you can substitute three cups of frozen corn.

Makes 6 servings

6 ears sweet corn
4 slices center-cut bacon, crisply
   cooked and crumbled
2 potatoes, peeled and diced
1/2 c. onion, chopped
1 red pepper, chopped
2 stalks celery, diced
2 c. low-sodium chicken broth
1/2 t. pepper
2 c. 2% reduced-fat milk
1 T. butter, sliced

Slice corn kernels from ears, reserving cobs. Place reserved cobs, corn kernels and remaining ingredients except milk and butter in a slow cooker. Cover and cook on high setting for 7 to 8 hours, until vegetables are tender. Remove corn cobs and discard. Purée half of soup using an immersion blender or food processor. Return puréed soup to slow cooker; stir in milk and butter. Cover and continue cooking on high setting until warmed through, about 15 to 30 minutes.

Nutrition Per Serving: 238 calories, 6g fat, 3g sat fat, 13mg cholesterol, 180mg sodium, 38g carbohydrate, 4g fiber, 11g protein

★ LOW-CAL ADD-ON ★ **Serve with 1/2 ounce of oyster crackers for an extra 60 calories.**

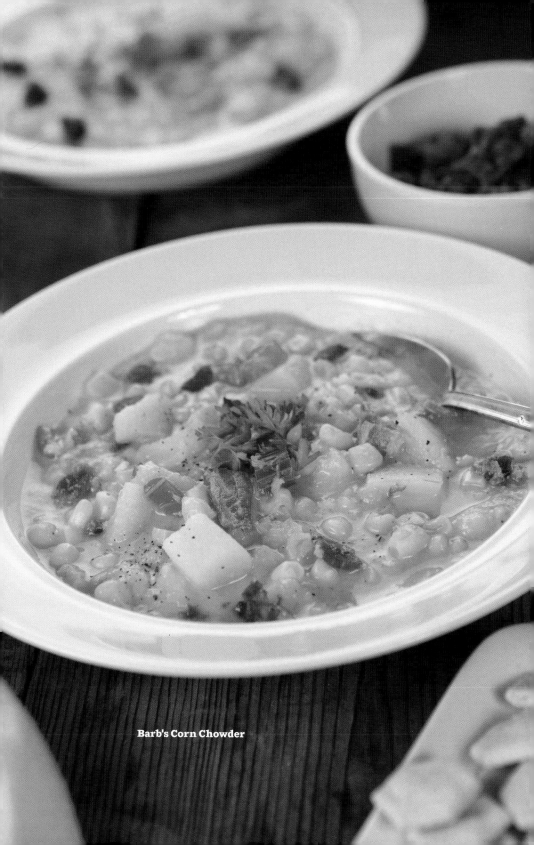

Barb's Corn Chowder

Sandy Coffey, Cincinnati, OH

Gram's Loaded Baked Potato Soup

Everyone loves baked potatoes, so this is a hearty meal in itself. Good on a chilly weekend day.

Makes 8 servings

32-oz. container low-sodium chicken broth
1/2 c. 2% reduced-fat milk
2 T. all-purpose flour
6 potatoes, peeled and diced
1/2 c. onion, chopped
1 t. salt
1 c. reduced-fat sour cream
8-oz. pkg. shredded reduced-fat Colby-Jack or mild Cheddar cheese
8 slices center-cut bacon, crisply cooked and crumbled

In a slow cooker, combine broth and milk. Whisk in flour; add potatoes, onion and salt. Cover and cook on low setting for 6 to 8 hours, until potatoes are tender. Stir in sour cream. Top individual servings with cheese and bacon.

Nutrition Per Serving: 307 calories, 8g fat, 5g sat fat,18 cholesterol, 631mg sodium, 44g carbohydrate, 4g fiber, 13g protein

Judy Sellgren, Wyoming, MI

Bacon & Wild Rice Soup

This smells great when I come home after a long day of work or shopping!

Makes 10 servings

10-oz. pkg. center-cut bacon, crisply cooked and crumbled
1 c. celery, chopped
1 onion, diced
12-oz. pkg. sliced mushrooms
1 c. cooked instant wild rice
2 10-3/4 oz. cans cream of mushroom soup
2 10-3/4 oz. cans cream of chicken soup
2 c. water
2 c. half-and-half

Combine all ingredients except half-and-half in slow cooker. Cover and cook on low setting for 8 to 10 hours, or on high setting for 4 to 6 hours. Stir in half-and-half 30 minutes before end of cooking time.

Nutrition Per Serving: 334 calories, 21g fat, 8g sat fat, 33mg cholesterol, 1303mg sodium, 16g carbohydrate, 21g fiber, 18g protein

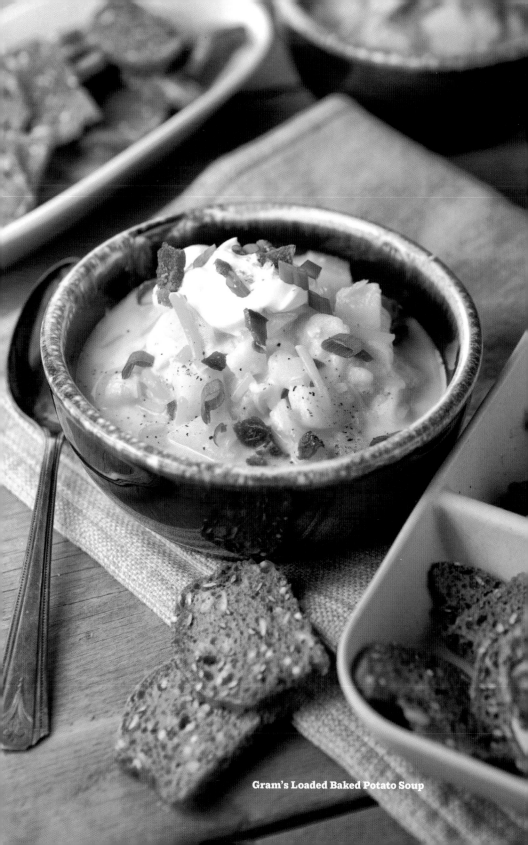

Gram's Loaded Baked Potato Soup

Darrell Lawry, Kissimmee, FL

Black Bean Chili

So good any time of year.

Makes 4 servings

1-lb. pork tenderloin

3 15-1/2 oz. cans black beans, drained
   and rinsed

16-oz. jar chunky salsa

1/2 c. low-sodium chicken broth

1 green pepper, chopped

1 onion, chopped

2 t. chili powder

1 t. ground cumin

1 t. dried oregano

Garnish: reduced-fat sour cream,
   diced tomatoes

Place pork in a lightly greased slow cooker; add remaining ingredients except garnish. Cover and cook on low setting for 8 hours, or on high setting for 4 hours. Shred pork; return to slow cooker. Garnish servings with dollops of sour cream and diced tomatoes.

Nutrition Per Serving: 326 calories, 3g fat, 1g sat fat, 74mg cholesterol, 1282mg sodium, 41g carbohydrate, 15g fiber, 35g protein

★ SAVVY SWAP ★ For a beefy option, make it with a lean sirloin roast instead the pork tenderloin.

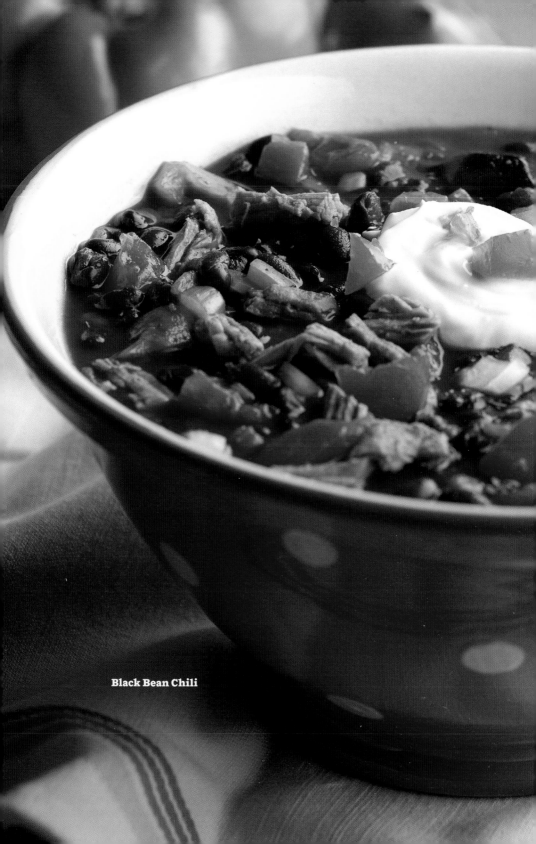

Black Bean Chili

SOUPS & STEWS

Lory Howard, Jackson, CA

Margaret's Lentil Soup

I received this hearty recipe from a great and fun friend of mine.

Makes 10 servings

1/4 c. olive oil
3 c. cooked lean ham, diced
1/2 lb. smoked turkey sausage links, sliced 1/2-inch thick
2 onions, chopped
1 clove garlic, pressed, or 1 t. garlic powder
12 c. water
3/4 lb. dried lentils, rinsed and sorted
2 c. celery with leaves, chopped
2 tomatoes, cut into wedges, or 14-1/2-oz. can whole tomatoes
10-oz. pkg. frozen cut leaf spinach, partially thawed
1-1/2 t. salt
1/2 t. hot pepper sauce

Heat oil in a skillet over medium heat. Add ham, sausage, onions and garlic. Cook for 5 minutes, stirring often. Drain; add to a slow cooker. Add remaining ingredients. Cover and cook on low setting for 8 to 10 hours, until lentils are tender. This soup freezes well.

Nutrition Per Serving: 340 calories, 15g fat, 4g sat fat, 53mg cholesterol, 642mg sodium, 27g carbohydrate, 6g fiber, 24g protein

Linda Neel, Lovington, NM

Green Chile Stew

Perfect for a cold evening! Use hot, medium or mild chiles, according to your own taste.

Makes 4 servings

1 lb. boneless pork, cubed
2 16-oz. cans pinto beans
2 14-1/2 oz. cans Mexican-style diced tomatoes
2 4-oz. cans diced green chiles
15-1/2 oz. can hominy, drained
1 t. ground cumin
pepper to taste

Place pork in a slow cooker. Top with remaining ingredients; stir. Cover and cook on high setting for 4 to 5 hours.

Nutrition Per Serving: 334 calories, 5g fat, 2g sat fat, 70mg cholesterol, 1330mg sodium, 37g carbohydrate, 10g fiber, 34g protein

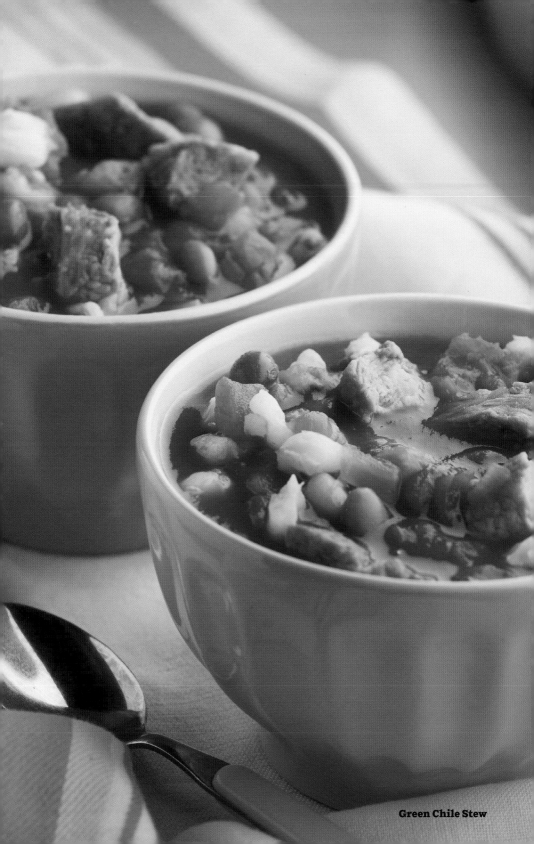

Green Chile Stew

Vickie, Gooseberry Patch

Zippy Chile Verde

This tangy pork dish is perfect served over steamed rice and black beans, or wrapped up in a tortilla with a little Pepper Jack cheese.

Makes 8 servings

3 T. olive oil
1/2 c. onion, chopped
2 cloves garlic, minced
3-lb. boneless pork shoulder, cubed
4 7-oz. cans green salsa
4-oz. can diced jalapeño peppers
14-1/2 oz. can no-salt diced tomatoes

Heat oil in a large skillet over medium heat. Add onion and garlic to oil; cook and stir until fragrant, about 2 minutes. Add pork to skillet; cook until browned on all sides. Transfer pork mixture to a slow cooker; stir in salsa, jalapeño peppers and tomatoes with juice. Cover and cook on high setting for 3 hours. Turn to low setting; cover and cook for 4 to 5 more hours.

Nutrition Per Serving: 332 calories, 16g total fat, 4g sat fat, 111mg cholesterol, 668 mg sodium, 10g carbohydrate, 1g fiber, 34g protein

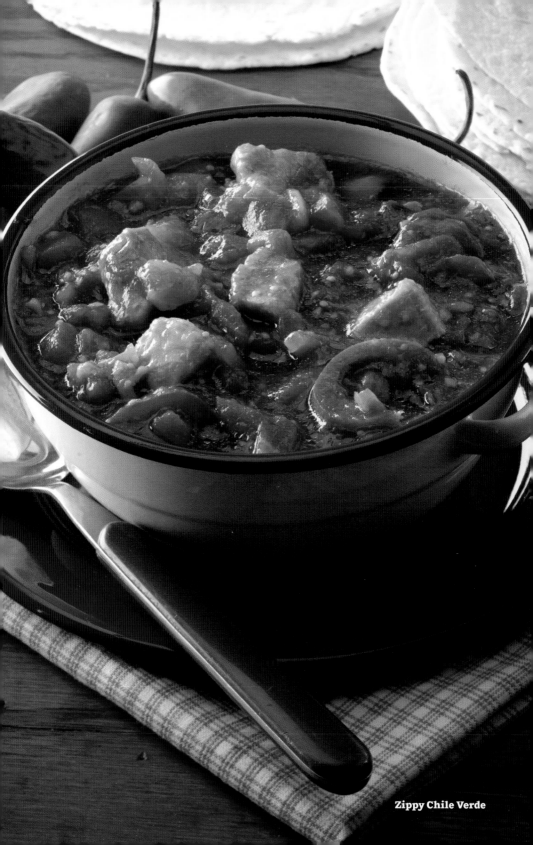

Zippy Chile Verde

Lorrie Smith, Drummonds, TN

Smoky White Bean Chili

I love white bean chili, but don't care for chicken, so I decided to try it with smoked sausages. Now I wouldn't make it any other way!

Makes 10 servings

5 15-1/2 oz. cans Great Northern
   beans, drained and rinsed
16-oz. pkg. mini smoked sausages
10-oz. can diced tomatoes with green
   chiles
1 T. dried, minced onion
1 T. chili powder
1/2 t. salt
1/2 t. pepper

Combine all ingredients in a slow cooker. Cover and cook on low setting for about 4 hours.

Nutrition Per Serving: 237 calories, 12g fat, 5g sat fat, 27mg cholesterol, 840mg sodium, 19g carbohydrate, 7g fiber, 13g protein

★ SAVVY SWAP ★ You can use a large smoked sausage and cut into slices instead of the mini variety.

Tori Willis, Champaign, IL

Southern BBQ Bean Soup

When my daughter visited Alabama, this was one recipe she brought home...it's become a family favorite up north too!

Makes 10 servings

1 lb. dried Great Northern beans, rinsed and sorted
3/4 c. onion, chopped
1/8 t. pepper
2 lbs. lean beef short ribs, cut into serving-size pieces
5 to 6 c. water
1 c. barbecue sauce
2 t. salt

In a large bowl, cover dried beans with water; soak for 8 hours to overnight. Drain beans, discarding water. Combine beans, onion, pepper and short ribs in a slow cooker; add 5 to 6 cups fresh water to cover. Cover and cook on low setting for 10 to 12 hours. Remove short ribs; cut meat from bones. Return meat to slow cooker; stir in barbecue sauce and salt to taste. Cover and cook on high setting for an additional 20 minutes, or until warmed through.

Nutrition Per Serving: 362 calories, 10g fat, 4g sat fat, 54mg cholesterol, 817mg sodium, 41g carbohydrate, 10g fiber, 28g protein

★ SAVVY SWAP ★ Sub dried navy beans for the Great Northern beans, if desired.

Jo Ann, Gooseberry Patch

Harvest Pork & Squash Stew

Try this flavorful stew on a fall day after the first snap of cold air. I like to serve it with warm sweet potato biscuits.

Makes 8 servings

1-1/2 lbs. pork shoulder roast, cubed and fat trimmed
1 t. salt
1 t. pepper
1 T. olive oil
1 onion, chopped
1-1/2 c. butternut squash, peeled and cubed
16-oz. pkg. baby carrots
8 new redskin potatoes, quartered
12-oz. jar homestyle pork gravy
1/4 c. water
1/4 c. catsup
1 t. dried sage
1/2 t. dried thyme

Season pork with salt and pepper. Heat oil in a large skillet over medium heat; add pork and onion. Cook, stirring often, until pork is browned all on all sides, about 5 minutes; drain. Combine pork mixture with remaining ingredients in a large slow cooker; stir gently. Cover and cook on low setting for 7 to 8 hours.

Nutrition Per Serving: 343 calories, 8g fat, 2g sat fat, 56mg cholesterol, 774mg sodium, 47g carbohydrate, 6g fiber, 23g protein

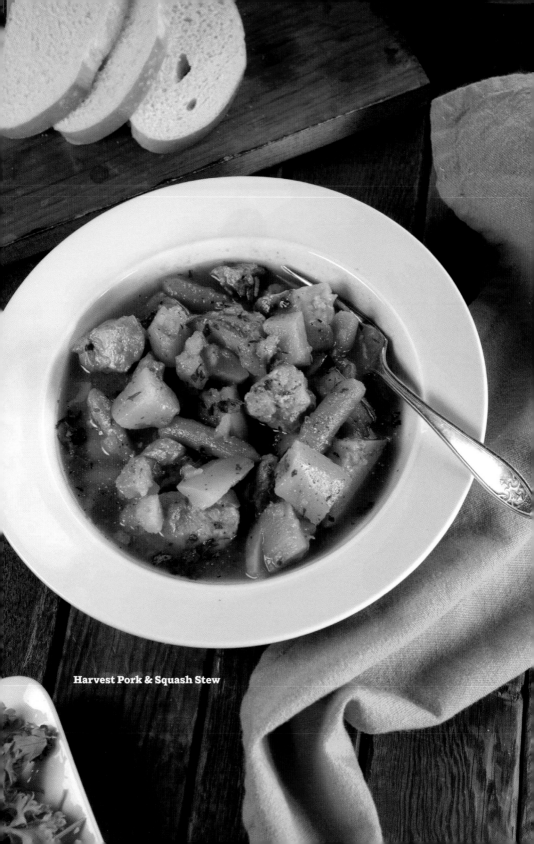

Harvest Pork & Squash Stew

Peggy Pelfrey, Fort Riley, KS

Chuck Wagon Stew

This hearty stew is ideal for a fall social or a weekend at the cabin.

Makes 8 servings

1-1/2 lbs. stew beef cubes
1/2 lb. smoked turkey sausage, sliced
1 onion, chopped
3 potatoes, peeled and cubed
28-oz. can barbecue baked beans

Place beef, sausage, onion and potatoes into a slow cooker; mix well. Spoon beans over top. Cover and cook on low setting for 8 to 10 hours, or on high setting for 4 to 5 hours. Stir again before serving.

Nutrition Per Serving: 344 calories, 8g fat, 3g sat fat, 72mg cholesterol, 732mg sodium, 40g carbohydrate, 6g fiber, 29g protein

Mel Chencharick, Julian, PA

Cider Pork Stew

This recipe gives the familiar taste of stew a new twist. Try it...it's very good!

Makes 8 servings

2 lbs. pork shoulder roast, cubed and fat trimmed
1 T. olive oil
3 potatoes, peeled and cut into 1/2-inch cubes
3 carrots, peeled and cut into 1/2-inch slices
2 onions, sliced
1/2 c. celery, coarsely chopped
2/3 c. apple, peeled, cored and coarsely chopped
2 c. apple cider or apple juice
3 T. quick-cooking tapioca, uncooked
1 t. caraway seed
1 t. salt
1/4 t. pepper
Optional: snipped fresh chives

Brown pork in oil in a large skillet over medium heat. Place pork in a 5-quart slow cooker. Add vegetables and apple; set aside. In a bowl, combine remaining ingredients except optional chives. Pour over pork mixture in slow cooker. Cover and cook on low setting for 10 to 12 hours, or on high setting for 5 to 6 hours, until pork is tender. If desired, top each serving with a sprinkle of snipped chives..

Nutrition Per Serving: 293 calories, 6g fat, 2g sat fat, 70mg cholesterol, 435mg sodium,33 carbohydrate, 3g fiber, 25g protein

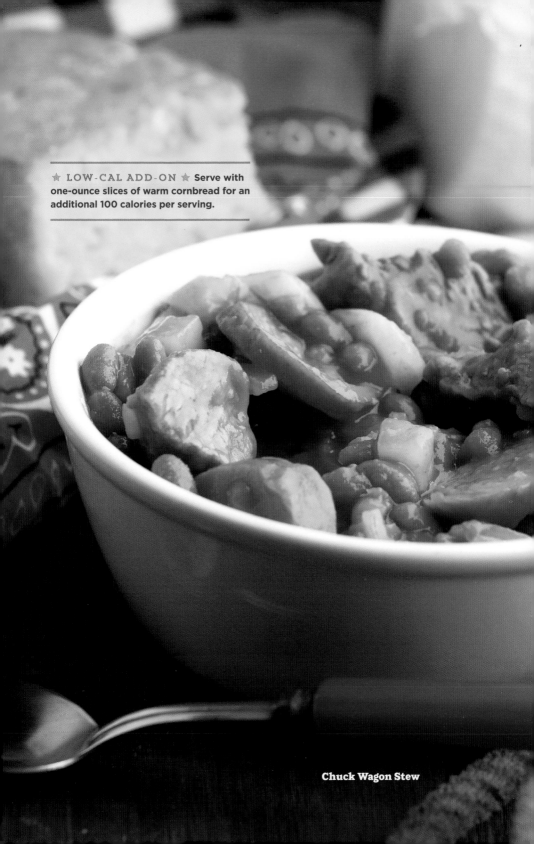

★ LOW-CAL ADD-ON ★ Serve with
one-ounce slices of warm cornbread for an
additional 100 calories per serving.

Chuck Wagon Stew

Marsha Baker, Pioneer, OH

Lightened-Up Cheeseburger Soup

This is a truly super soup! I combined ideas from two recipes to make this one comforting dish. And I've used lighter ingredients, but only you will know that!

Makes 8 servings

1 T. olive oil
1 onion, chopped
1 stalk celery, chopped
1 clove garlic, minced
1 lb. lean ground beef
3 T. all-purpose flour
3 c. low-sodium chicken broth, divided
15-oz. can fire-roasted diced tomatoes, partially drained
1 c. 2% reduced-fat evaporated milk
8-oz. pkg. reduced-fat pasteurized process cheese, cubed
1/2 t. paprika
1/4 t. salt
1/4 t. pepper
Garnish: baked tortilla chips, crushed

Add oil to a Dutch oven; heat over medium-high heat for 30 seconds. Add onion, celery and garlic. Cook, stirring often, until tender, 5 to 10 minutes. Coat a 4-quart slow cooker with non-stick vegetable spray; spoon in onion mixture and set aside. In the same skillet, brown beef over medium-heat, breaking up beef as it cooks. Drain and add beef to slow cooker. In a small cup, combine flour and 1/2 cup broth; stir until smooth and lump-free. Pour flour mixture into same skillet; add remaining broth. Bring to a simmer, scraping up any browned bits in bottom of skillet; pour into slow cooker. Stir in remaining ingredients except tortilla chips. Cover and cook on low setting for 2 hours. Serve soup topped with crushed chips.

Nutrition Per Serving: 223 calories, 9g fat, 4g sat fat, 53mg cholesterol, 658mg sodium, 13g carbohydrate, 1g fiber, 21g protein

---

★ LOW-CAL ADD-ON ★ **Enjoy the baked tortilla chips in your soup without the guilt! One serving of tortilla chips (about 16 chips) has 120 calories.**

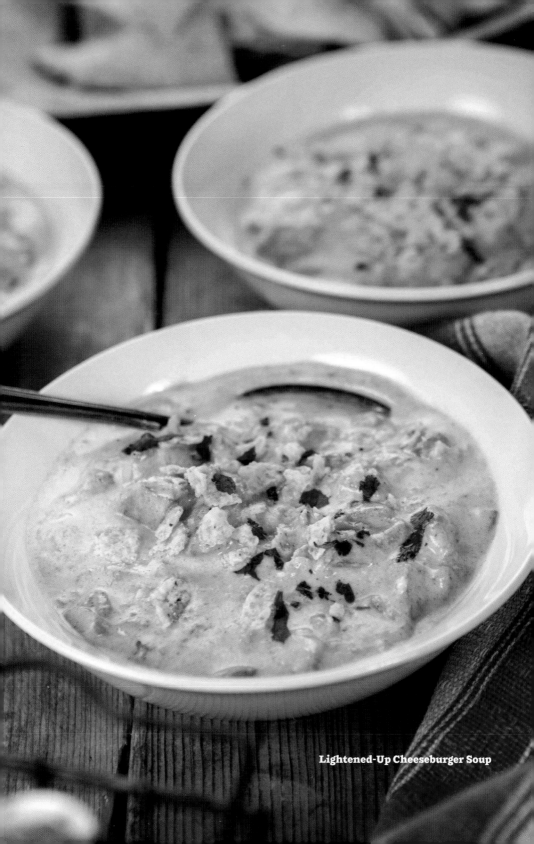

Lightened-Up Cheeseburger Soup

Cami Cherryholmes, Urbana, IA

Vegetable Beef Soup

This recipe is as good-tasting as it is easy...it also freezes well.

Makes 6 servings

1 lb. lean ground beef, browned and drained
16-oz. pkg. frozen mixed vegetables
12-oz. can cocktail vegetable juice
3 c. water
1/2 c. pearled barley
1-1/2 oz. pkg. onion soup mix
3 cubes beef bouillon

Combine all ingredients in a slow cooker; cook on low setting for 6 to 8 hours.

Nutrition Per Serving: 227 calories, 8g fat, 2g sat fat, 48mg cholesterol, 1042mg sodium, 20g carbohydrate, 5g fiber, 21g protein

Lynn McKaige, Savage, MN

Beef Barley Soup

Makes 6 servings

2 c. carrots, peeled and thinly sliced
1 c. celery, thinly sliced
3/4 c. red or green pepper, diced
1 c. onion, diced
1 lb. stew beef cubes
1/2 c. pearl barley, uncooked
1/4 c. fresh parsley, chopped
3 cubes beef bouillon
2 T. catsup
1 t. salt
3/4 t. dried basil
5 c. water

Layer vegetables, beef and barley in a slow cooker; add remaining ingredients except water. Pour water over all; do not stir. Cover and cook low setting for 9 to 11 hours.

Nutrition Per Serving: 384 calories, 4g fat, 2g sat fat, 49mg cholesterol, 978mg sodium, 66g carbohydrate, 10g fiber, 25g protein

★ SAVVY SWAP ★ Use 5 cups of low-sodium beef broth instead of the beef bouillon and water, if you like.

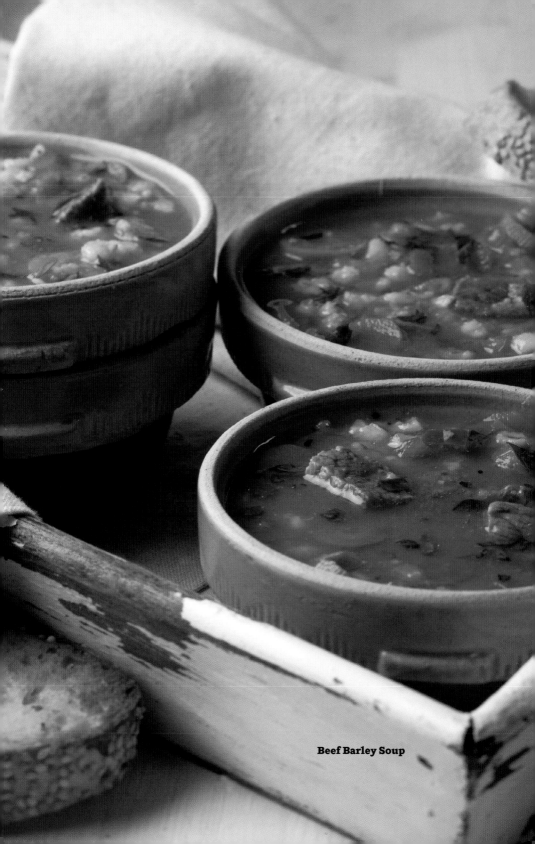

Beef Barley Soup

Marla Kinnersley, Littleton, CO

Pasta Fagioli Soup

This is one of my favorite go-to soups! I make it often for Sunday dinners and then we have leftovers for busy Mondays. It is very satisfying served with bread sticks and a crisp tossed salad.

Makes 8 servings

1 lb. lean ground beef
1 yellow onion, chopped
14-1/2 oz. can diced tomatoes
26-oz. jar spaghetti sauce
3-1/2 c. low-sodium beef broth
15-1/2 oz. can kidney beans, drained
   and rinsed
1 c. carrots, peeled and grated
1 c. celery, sliced
1 T. white balsamic vinegar
1 t. dried basil
1 t. dried oregano
1/2 t. dried thyme
1/2 t. pepper
1/2 t. hot pepper sauce
1-1/2 c. small shell pasta, uncooked
2 t. fresh parsley, chopped

In a skillet over medium heat, brown beef with onion. Drain; add beef mixture to a 5-quart slow cooker. Add tomatoes with juice and remaining ingredients except pasta and parsley; stir. Cover and cook on low setting for 7 to 8 hours. About 15 minutes before serving, stir in uncooked pasta and parsley. Cover and cook on low setting for 15 minutes more, or until pasta is tender.

Nutrition Per Serving: 220 calories, 6g fat, 2g sat fat, 40mg cholesterol, 700mg sodium, 23g carbohydrate, 5g fiber, 17g protein

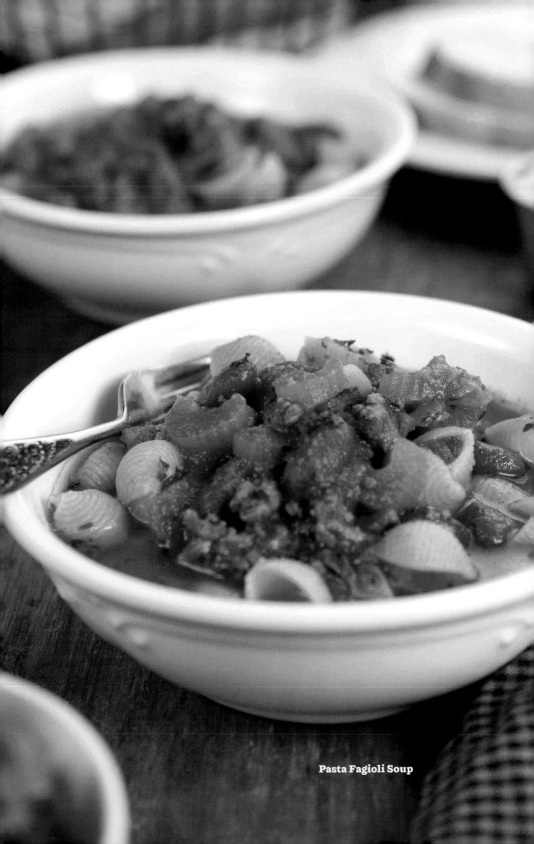

Pasta Fagioli Soup

Karen Wilson, Defiance, OH

Weeknight Beef Stew

A hearty recipe that's easy to toss together.

Makes 8 servings

2 lbs. stew beef cubes
1-3/4 c. low-sodium beef broth
11-1/2 oz. can vegetable cocktail juice
4 potatoes, peeled and cubed
2 stalks celery, chopped
2 carrots, peeled and chopped
1 sweet onion, chopped
3 bay leaves
1/2 t. dried thyme
1/2 t. chili powder
1 t. salt
1/4 t. pepper
2 T. cornstarch
1 T. cold water
1/2 c. frozen peas
1/2 c. frozen corn

In a large slow cooker, combine all ingredients except cornstarch, cold water, peas and corn. Cover and cook on low setting for 7 to 8 hours, until beef is tender. Discard bay leaves. In a small bowl, stir together cornstarch and cold water until smooth. Stir mixture into stew; add corn and peas. Cook on high setting for 30 minutes, or until thickened.

Nutrition Per Serving: 277 calories, 6g fat, 2g sat fat, 73mg cholesterol, 518mg sodium, 28 carbohydrate, 3g fiber, 28g protein

Audrey Laudenat, East Haddam, CT

Divine Seafood Chowder

This hearty chowder is a meal all in itself! Be sure to pass a basket of oyster crackers.

Makes 6 servings

1 onion, sliced
4 potatoes, peeled and sliced
2 t. garlic, minced
1 t. dill weed
2 T. butter
1 c. bottled clam juice, heated
   to boiling
15-oz. can creamed corn
1 t. salt
1 t. pepper
1/2 lb. haddock or cod fillet
1/2 lb. uncooked medium shrimp,
   peeled and halved
1 c. light cream, warmed

Layer all ingredients except cream in a slow cooker, placing fish and shrimp on top. Cover and cook on high setting for one hour; reduce setting to low and cook for 3 hours. Just before serving, gently stir in cream.

Nutrition Per Serving: 360 calories, 18g fat, 10g sat fat, 123mg cholesterol, 858mg sodium, 36g carbohydrate, 3g fiber, 16g protein

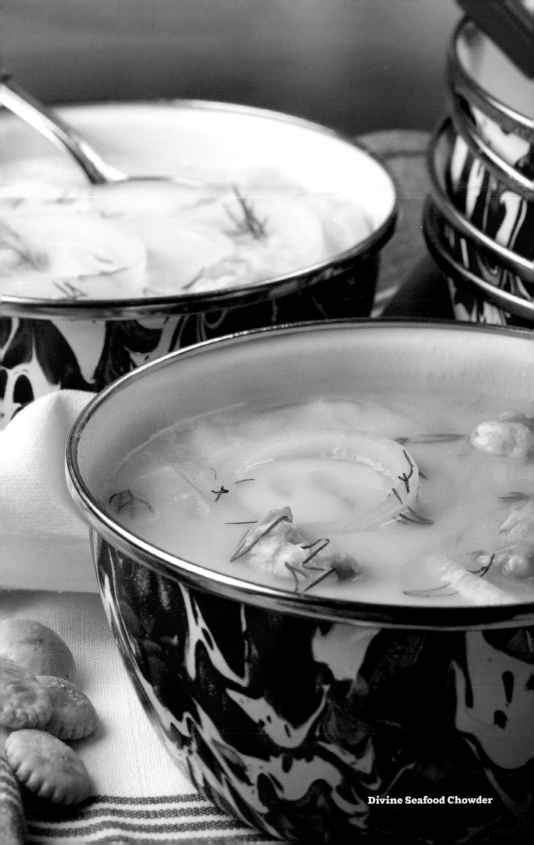

Divine Seafood Chowder

Erin Kelly, Jefferson City, MO

Turkey Noodle Soup

My mom and I first made this recipe for dinner after going to a fall festival. It was a warm and delicious end to a great day with her, and a good way to use up leftover turkey!

Makes 6 servings

5 c. low-sodium chicken broth
10-3/4 oz. can cream of chicken soup
15-oz. can corn, drained
1 t. salt
1 t. pepper
1/2 c. onion, finely chopped
1/2 c. green onions, sliced
1/2 c. carrot, peeled and finely chopped
1/2 c. celery, finely chopped
1-1/2 c. medium egg noodles, uncooked
2 c. cooked turkey, chopped

In a slow cooker, combine all ingredients except noodles and turkey. Cover and cook on low setting for 4 to 5 hours. Stir in noodles and turkey. Turn slow cooker to high setting; cover and cook for one additional hour.

Nutrition Per Serving: 317 calories, 13 fat, 3g sat fat, 98mg cholesterol, 953mg sodium, 22g carbohydrate, 4g fiber, 27g protein

★ SAVVY SWAP ★ To save time, use pre-chopped onion and celery from your supermarket's produce section.

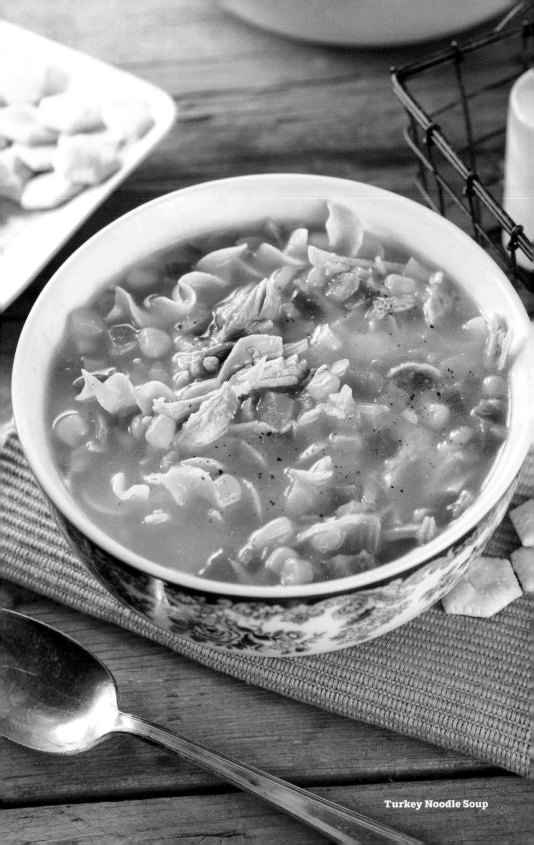

Turkey Noodle Soup

Shannon O'Donnell, East Wilton, ME

New England Chili

Great served over rice, in bread bowls or with cornbread. Garnish with shredded Cheddar cheese and sour cream.

Makes 10 servings

2 lbs. ground turkey, browned and drained
1 onion, chopped
28-oz. can diced tomatoes
2 8-oz. cans tomato purée
2 16-oz. cans kidney beans
4-oz. can diced green chiles
1 t. garlic, minced
2 to 3 T. chili powder
1-1/2 t. salt
1 t. pepper

Spray a slow cooker with non-stick vegetable spray. Combine all ingredients in slow cooker. Cover and cook on low setting for 4 to 6 hours.

Nutrition Per Serving: 242 calories, 8g fat, 2g sat fat, 67mg cholesterol, 825mg sodium, 20g carbohydrate, 5g fiber, 23g protein

Janet Allen, Houser, ID

Chicken Taco Soup

A spicy and flavorful soup...serve this favorite with bandannas for napkins and a bottle of hot pepper sauce for those who like it fiery!

Makes 8 servings

1 onion, chopped
16-oz. can chili beans, drained
15-oz. can black beans, drained and rinsed
15-oz. can corn, drained
2 10-oz. cans diced tomatoes with green chiles
8-oz. can tomato sauce
12-oz. can regular or non-alcoholic beer
1-1/4 oz. pkg. less-sodium taco seasoning mix
3 6-oz. boneless, skinless chicken breasts
Optional: shredded reduced-fat Cheddar cheese, crushed tortilla chips, reduced-fat sour cream

In a slow cooker, mix together onion, beans, corn, diced tomatoes with juice, tomato sauce and beer. Add seasoning mix; stir to blend. Lightly press chicken breasts into mixture in slow cooker until partially covered. Cover and cook on low setting for 5 hours. Remove chicken from slow cooker; shred and return to soup. Cover and cook for an additional 2 hours. Top servings of soup with cheese, crushed chips and sour cream, if desired.

Nutrition Per Serving: 262 calories, 3g fat, 1g sat fat, 62mg cholesterol, 1273mg sodium, 28g carbohydrate, 7g fiber, 25g protein

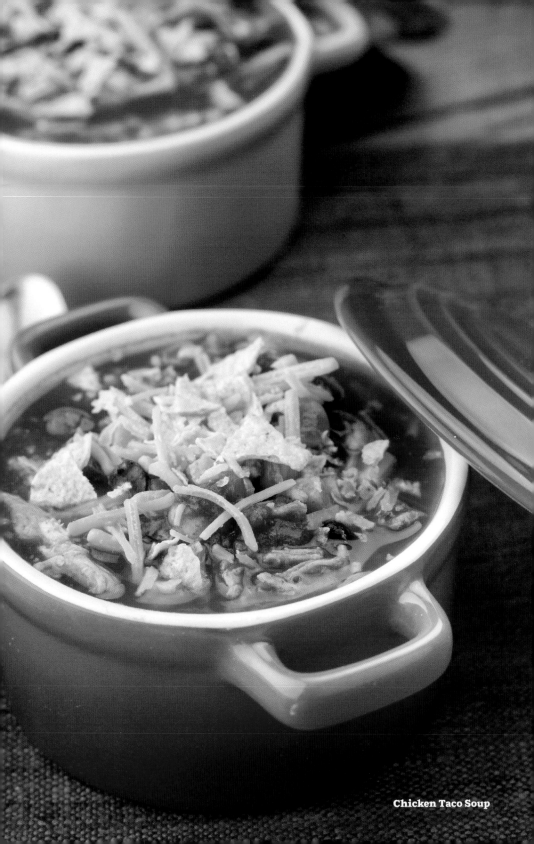

Chicken Taco Soup

Linda Belon, Winterville, OH

Winter Vegetable Stew

A scrumptious chunky meatless stew... perfect for snow-day lunches and chilly tailgating parties.

Makes 4 servings

28-oz. can Italian peeled whole
   tomatoes, drained and liquid
   reserved
14-1/2 oz. can low-sodium vegetable
   or chicken broth
4 redskin potatoes, cut into 1/2-inch
   cubes
2 c. celery, cut into 1/2-inch slices
1-1/2 c. carrots, peeled and cut into
   1/2-inch slices
1 c. parsnips, peeled and cut into
   1/2-inch slices
2 leeks, cut into 1/2-inch slices
1/2 t. salt
1/2 t. dried thyme
1/2 t. dried rosemary
3 T. cornstarch
3 T. cold water

Coarsely chop tomatoes and add to a 5-quart slow cooker along with reserved liquid. Add remaining ingredients except cornstarch and cold water. Cover and cook on low setting for 8 to 10 hours. About 30 minutes before serving, dissolve cornstarch in cold water; gradually stir into stew until well blended. Cover and cook on high setting about 20 minutes, stirring occasionally, until thickened.

Nutrition Per Serving: 307 calories, 1g fat, 0g sat fat, 0mg cholesterol, 824mg sodium, 69g carbohydrate, 12g fiber, 8g protein

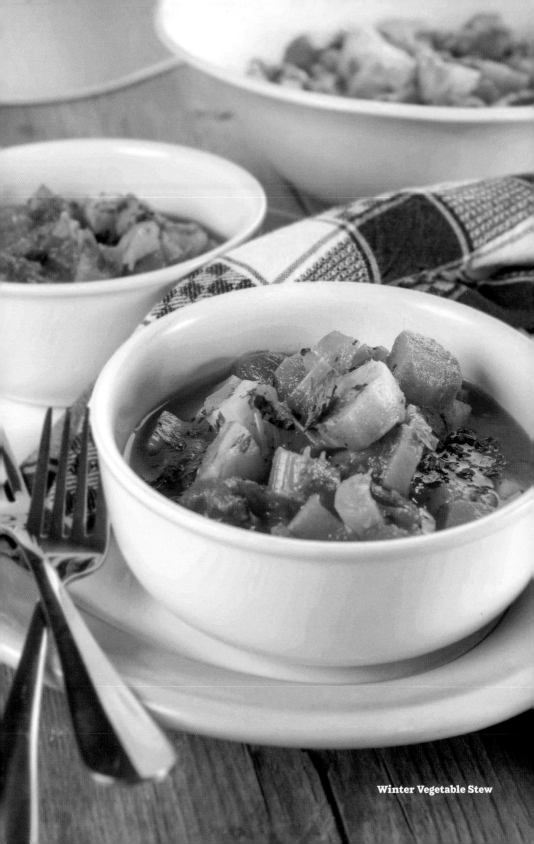

Winter Vegetable Stew

Gladys Brehm, Quakertown, PA

Easy Vegetable Soup

Quick & easy...a very satisfying meal on cold days.

Makes 6 servings

64-oz. can cocktail vegetable juice
32-oz. pkg. frozen mixed vegetables
2 c. cooked lean ground beef or
   chicken, chopped
1 c. curly pasta or small shell pasta,
   uncooked

Combine all ingredients in a 5-quart slow cooker. Cover and cook on high setting for 3 to 4 hours, stirring occasionally.

Nutrition Per Serving: 296 calories, 6g fat, 3g sat fat, 48mg cholesterol, 708mg sodium, 30g carbohydrate, 8g fiber, 27g protein

★ SAVVY SWAP ★ You can also use elbow macaroni in this cozy soup.

Penny Sherman, Ava, MO

Garden-Style Navy Bean Soup

We love old-fashioned bean and ham soup, but this soup with spicy tomatoes and spinach is fresh tasting and different. Use plain diced tomatoes, if you prefer a milder flavor.

Makes 8 servings

1 lb. dried navy beans, rinsed and sorted
6 c. water
14-1/2 oz. can diced tomatoes with spicy red pepper
2 c. cooked lean ham, diced
1 onion, chopped
3 stalks celery, thinly sliced
3 carrots, peeled and thinly sliced
1/2 t. dried thyme
1 t. salt
1/4 t. pepper
5-oz. pkg. baby spinach

In a large bowl, cover dried beans with water; soak for 8 hours to overnight. Drain beans, discarding water. Add beans to a slow cooker. Stir in 6 cups fresh water, tomatoes with juice and remaining ingredients except salt, pepper and spinach. Cover and cook on low setting for 9 to 10 hours, until beans are tender. Remove 2 cups of soup to a blender. Process until puréed; return to slow cooker. Add salt and pepper; gradually add spinach and stir until wilted.

Nutrition Per Serving: 297 calories, 4g fat, 1g sat fat, 32mg cholesterol, 480mg sodium, 42g carbohydrate, 11g fiber, 24 protein

---

★ LOW-CAL ADD-ON ★ **Serve with baguette toasts to dip in the soup. A one-ounce serving has 100 calories.**

Marie Matter, Dallas, TX

Vegetarian Quinoa Chili

This hearty chili couldn't be easier. Just combine everything in your slow cooker, and hours later you'll have a healthy, tasty meal that everyone in your family will love. Enjoy!

Makes 6 servings

2 14-1/2 oz. cans diced tomatoes with green chiles
15-oz. can tomato sauce
15-oz. can kidney beans, drained and rinsed
15-oz. can black beans, drained and rinsed
1-1/2 c. low-sodium vegetable broth
1 c. frozen corn
1 c. quinoa, uncooked and rinsed
1 onion, diced
3 cloves garlic, minced
2 T. chili powder
2 t. ground cumin

1-1/2 t. smoked paprika
1-1/2 t. sugar
1/4 t. cayenne pepper
1/2 t. ground coriander
1/2 t. kosher salt
1/4 t. pepper
Garnish: shredded Cheddar cheese, sour cream, sliced avocado, chopped fresh cilantro

Combine undrained tomatoes and remaining ingredients except garnish in a slow cooker; stir together. Cover and cook on low setting for 6 to 8 hours, or on high setting for 3 to 4 hours. To serve, ladle into soup bowls; garnish as desired.

Nutrition Per Serving: 270 calories, 3g fat, 0g sat fat, 0mg cholesterol, 1185mg sodium, 51g carbohydrate, 11g fiber, 13g protein

★ LOW-CAL ADD-ON ★ **Top each soup serving with one tablespoon cheese, one tablespoon sour cream and 2 slices of avocado for an extra 120 calories.**

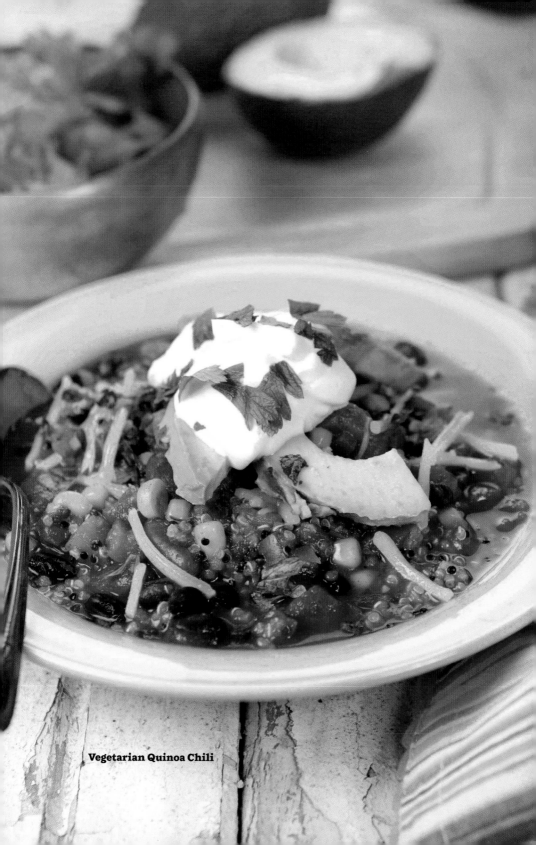

Vegetarian Quinoa Chili

Robin Hill, Rochester, NY

French Onion Soup

Now you can enjoy this elegant soup any time and it's so easy to prepare.

Makes 6 servings

1/4 c. butter

3 c. onions, sliced

1 T. sugar

1 t. salt

2 T. all-purpose flour

4 c. low-sodium beef broth

1/4 c. dry white wine or low-sodium beef broth

6 1-oz. slices French bread

1/2 c. grated Parmesan cheese

1/2 c. shredded part-skim mozzarella cheese

Melt butter in a large skillet over medium heat. Add onions; cook for 15 to 20 minutes, until soft. Stir in sugar and salt; continue to cook and stir until golden. Add flour; mix well. Combine onion mixture, broth and wine or broth in a slow cooker. Cover and cook on high setting for 3 to 4 hours. Ladle soup into oven-proof bowls. Top with bread slices; sprinkle with cheeses. Broil until cheese is bubbly and melted.

Nutrition Per Serving: 271 calories, 13g fat, 7g sat fat, 34mg cholesterol, 902mg sodium, 29g carbohydrate, 2 fiber, 9g protein

Jess Brunink, Whitehall, MI

Jess's Vegan Pea Soup

My version of pea soup...I love this stuff! It's cheap, filling and will feed a large family. I have four kiddos and a husband and we all love it! When we have leftovers, I even eat it for breakfast. If you are not vegan, a little sliced turkey or ham included is also really tasty.

Makes 10 servings

2 lbs. dried split peas, rinsed and sorted
8 c. water
3 cloves garlic, minced
3 potatoes, peeled and diced
1 onion, diced
1 t. salt

Combine all ingredients in a slow cooker; stir gently. Cover and cover on low setting for 8 hours, or until peas are tender.

Nutrition Per Serving: 318 calories, 1g fat, 0g sat fat, 0mg cholesterol, 246mg sodium, 60g carbohydrate, 20g fiber, 20g protein

★ LOW-CAL ADD-ON ★ Serve with a simple salad made with a package of herb salad mix, carrot ribbons and sliced onion drizzled with balsamic vinaigrette.

Glenn Stracqualursi, Lakeland, FL

Dad's Famous Minestrone

This one's in honor of my dad. For years, he made this tasty soup at his park's fundraiser events and never had any left by the end.

Serves 10

4 carrots, peeled and sliced
1 c. celery, chopped
1 c. onion, chopped
5 to 6 redskin potatoes, diced
3 zucchini, sliced
14-1/2 oz. can no-salt diced tomatoes
15-oz. can cut green beans
8 cloves garlic, chopped
3 T. olive oil
1-1/2 t. dried basil
1 t. dried rosemary
2 T. dried parsley
1/2 t. sea salt
1/2 t. pepper
3 14-oz. cans low-sodium chicken broth
12-oz. bottle cocktail vegetable juice
1 bunch fresh escarole, chopped
15-oz. can low-sodium garbanzo beans
15-oz. can low-sodium cannellini beans
8-oz. pkg. ditalini pasta, uncooked
Garnish: grated Parmesan cheese

To a slow cooker, add all ingredients in order listed except beans, pasta and garnish. Cover and cook on low setting for 8 hours. After 8 hours, stir in beans and uncooked pasta; cook for one more hour. Top servings with cheese.

Nutrition Per Serving: 328 calories, 6g total fat, 1g sat fat, 0mg cholesterol, 460 mg sodium, 60g carbohydrate, 11g fiber, 14g protein

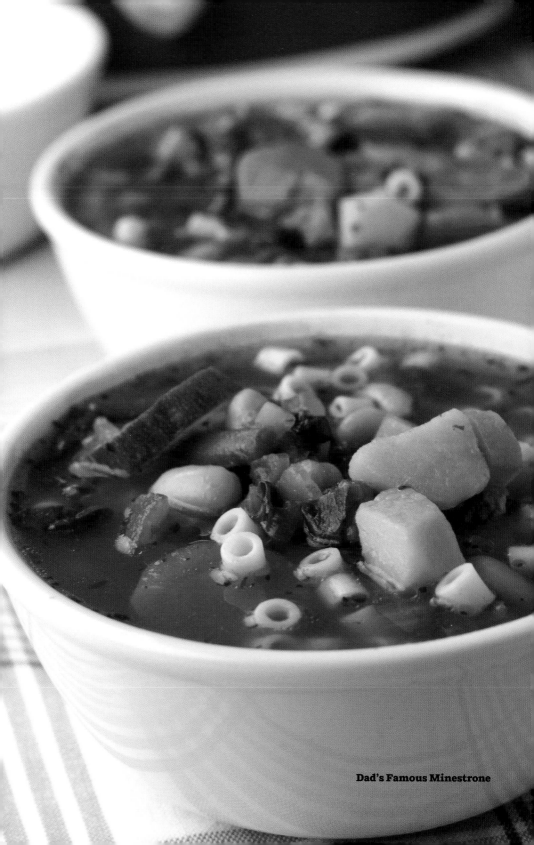

Dad's Famous Minestrone

Marcia Shaffer, Conneaut Lake, PA

French Lentil Soup

My great-great-grandmother was from France. This is a very old recipe passed down through many generations.

Makes 8 servings

6 T. olive oil
1 onion, chopped
2 cloves garlic, minced
12 c. water
1-1/2 c. dried lentils, rinsed and sorted
1 potato, peeled and diced
1 stalk celery, finely chopped
1 turnip, peeled and diced
1 carrot, peeled and finely chopped
1 c. tomato sauce
1 t. salt
1 t. pepper
1 bay leaf
1 bunch fresh sorrel or spinach, torn
1/2 c. cooked brown rice

Heat oil in a skillet over medium heat. Add onion and cook until soft, about 5 minutes. Add garlic; cook 3 minutes. Add onion mixture and remaining ingredients except sorrel or spinach and rice to a slow cooker. Cover and cook on low setting for 8 hours. Discard bay leaf. Shortly before serving time, add sorrel or spinach and cooked rice to slow cooker. Cover and cook for several minutes, until greens wilt; stir well.

Nutrition Per Serving: 281 calories, 11g fat, 2g sat fat, 0mg cholesterol, 488mg sodium, 37g carbohydrate, 6g fiber, 11g protein

★ SAVVY SWAP ★ Fresh kale would also make a good sub for the sorrel.

Amanda Black, Carterville, GA

Chili Sans Carne

At my local ladies' gym, we had a challenge to create a recipe that was high in healthy flavor and low in salt. I adapted my old meat-and-fat-filled recipe to make it healthier and meatless...it's a winner!

Makes 4 servings

2 15-oz. cans no-sodium-added black
   beans, drained and rinsed
15-oz. can no-sodium-added kidney
   beans, drained and rinsed
15-oz. can corn, drained and rinsed
14-1/2 oz. can diced tomatoes
6-oz. can tomato paste
1/2 c. onion, chopped
Garnish: thinly sliced green onions,
   low-sodium whole-wheat crackers

Combine beans and corn in a slow cooker. Add tomatoes with juice, tomato paste, onion and garlic. Cover and cook on low setting for 7 to 8 hours. Garnish with green onions; serve with crackers.

Nutrition Per Serving: 282 calories, 2g fat, 0g sat fat, 0mg cholesterol, 684mg sodium, 51g carbohydrate, 16 fiber, 15g protein

---

★ SAVVY SWAP ★ Use pinto beans instead of the black beans, if desired.

Jo Ann, Gooseberry Patch

Pumpkin Patch Soup

Every fall, my family begs me to make this soup. They like it so much, I've started making it year 'round!

Makes 6 servings

2 t. olive oil
1/2 c. raw pumpkin seeds
3 slices thick-cut bacon
1 onion, chopped
1/2 t. salt
1/2 t. chipotle powder
1/2 t. pepper
2 29-oz. cans pumpkin
4 c. low-sodium chicken broth
3/4 c. apple cider
1/2 c. whole milk

Heat oil in a small skillet over medium heat. Add pumpkin seeds to oil; cook and stir until seeds begin to pop, about one minute. Remove seeds to a bowl and set aside. Add bacon to skillet and cook until crisp. Remove bacon to a paper towel; crumble and refrigerate. Add onion to drippings in pan. Sauté until translucent, about 5 minutes. Stir in seasonings. Spoon onion mixture into a slow cooker. Whisk pumpkin, broth and cider into onion mixture. Cover and cook on high setting for 4 hours. Whisk in milk. Top servings with pumpkin seeds and crumbled bacon.

Nutrition Per Serving: 238 calories, 10g fat, 3g sat fat, 12mg cholesterol, 573mg sodium, 32g carbohydrate, 9g fiber, 8g protein

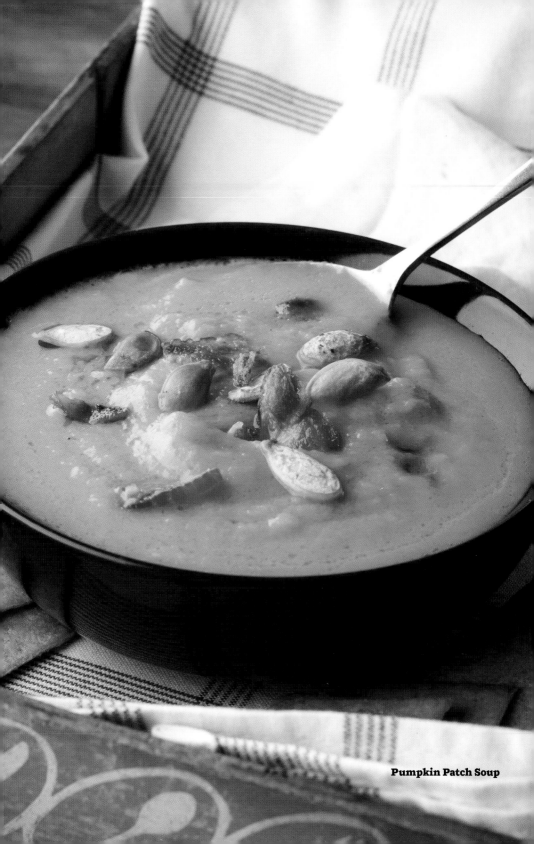

Pumpkin Patch Soup

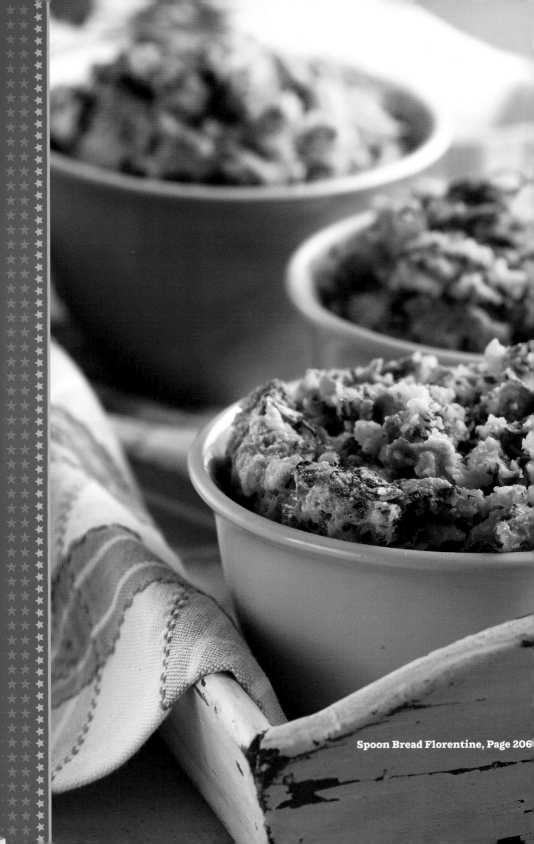

Spoon Bread Florentine, Page 206

CHAPTER SEVEN

Sides

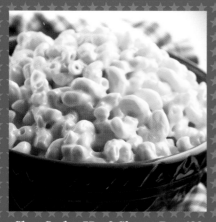

Slow-Cooker Mac & Cheese, Page 198

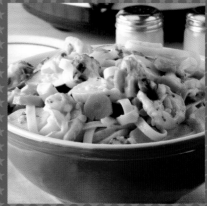

Garden-Style Fettuccine, Page 196

SIDES

Angela Murphy, Tempe AZ

Dijon-Ginger Carrots

Tangy mustard and ginger, sweet
brown sugar...I just adore this
super-simple dressed-up carrot recipe!
Garnish with snipped fresh chives
or mint.

Makes 12 servings

**12 carrots, peeled and sliced 1/4-inch
    thick
1/3 c. Dijon mustard
1/2 c. brown sugar, packed
1 t. fresh ginger, peeled and minced
1/4 t. salt
1/8 t. pepper**

Combine all ingredients in a slow
cooker; stir. Cover and cook on high
setting for 2 to 3 hours, until carrots are
tender, stirring twice during cooking.

Nutrition Per Serving: 71 calories, 0g fat, 0g
sat fat, 0mg cholesterol, 261mg sodium, 16
carbohydrate, 2g fiber, 1g protein

★ SAVVY SWAP ★ **Use honey instead of
brown sugar, if desired.**

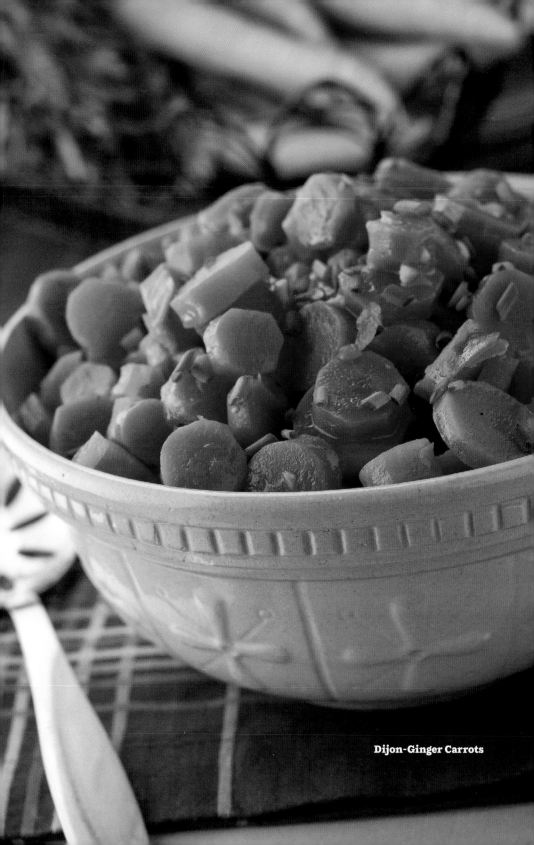

Dijon-Ginger Carrots

Karen Dennis, Mount Vernon, OH

Schnitzel Beans

My mom used to make this for our family get-togethers. She says the recipe was probably first used by my great-grandma. You'll know it's the right amount of vinegar when your eyes water!

Makes 8 servings

1/4 lb. center-cut bacon
1 onion, chopped
1/2 c. sugar
1/4 c. to 1/2 c. cider vinegar
8 c. fresh green beans, trimmed

In a skillet over medium heat, cook bacon until crisp. Drain and refrigerate bacon, reserving drippings in skillet. Allow drippings to cool slightly; add onion, sugar and 1/4 cup vinegar. Cook until sugar is dissolved, onion is tender and vinegar aroma is strong. Transfer beans to a slow cooker; cover with vinegar mixture. Add remaining vinegar, if desired. Cover and cook on low setting for 4 to 5 hours, or on high setting for 2 to 3 hours. Garnish with reserved bacon.

Nutrition Per Serving: 152 calories, 4g total fat, 2g sat fat, 5mg cholesterol, 236mg sodium, 21g carbohydrate, 3g fiber, 9g protein

Lisa Ann Panzino-DiNunzio, Vineland, NJ

Parsley Buttered Potatoes

Butter, chives and a dash of lemon juice jump-start this super-easy, super tasty recipe. These potatoes are perfect for toting to a potluck or get-together.

Makes 6 servings

1-1/2 lbs. new redskin potatoes
1/4 c. water
1/4 c. butter, melted
1 T. lemon juice
3 T. fresh parsley, minced
1 T. fresh chives, snipped
1/2 t. salt
1/2 t. pepper

If desired, pare a strip around the middle of each potato. Place potatoes and water in a slow cooker. Cover and cook on high setting for 2-1/2 to 3 hours, until tender; drain. In a small bowl, combine butter, lemon juice, parsley and chives. Pour over potatoes to coat. Sprinkle with salt and pepper.

Nutrition Per Serving: 145 calories, 8g total fat, 5g sat fat, 20mg cholesterol, 275mg sodium, 18g carbohydrate, 2g fiber, 2g protein

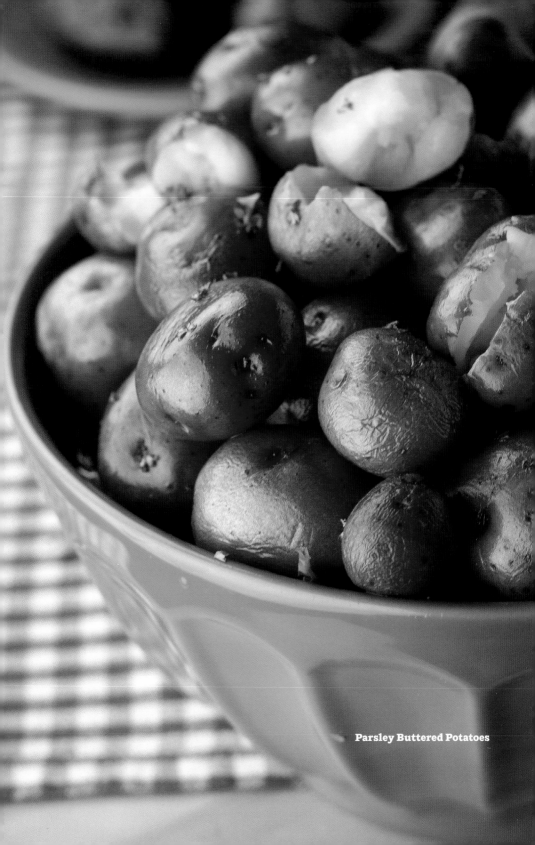

Parsley Buttered Potatoes

Lisa Ann Panzino-DiNunzio,
Vineland, NJ

Chunky Applesauce

There's nothing like homemade applesauce, and it can't get any easier than this yummy slow-cooker version. Some great apples for this recipe are Fuji, Golden Delicious and Gala.

Makes 8 servings

10 apples, peeled, cored and cubed
1/2 c. water
1/4 c. sugar
Optional: 1 t. cinnamon

Combine all ingredients in a slow cooker; toss to mix. Cover and cook on low setting for 8 to 10 hours. Serve warm or keep refrigerated in a covered container.

Nutrition Per Serving: 121 calories, 0g total fat, 0g sat fat, 0mg cholesterol, 0mg sodium, 32g carbohydrate, 3g fiber, 1 g protein

Megan Brooks, Antioch, TN

Sweet-and-Sour Red Cabbage

My Grandma Studer used to make a version of this. It's an old-fashioned side that's good with grilled sausages.

Makes 8 servings

4 slices center-cut bacon, diced
1/4 c. brown sugar, packed
2 T. all-purpose flour
1/4 c. cider vinegar
1/4 c. water
1/2 t. salt
1/8 t. pepper
1 head red cabbage, shredded
1/4 c. onion, finely chopped

In a skillet over medium heat, cook bacon until crisp. Drain and refrigerate bacon, reserving one tablespoon drippings. In a bowl, combined reserved drippings, flour, vinegar, water and seasonings; stir until smooth. Place cabbage and onion in a slow cooker. Pour mixture over top; toss to mix well. Cover and cook on low setting for 6 to 7 hours, until cabbage is tender. Serve warm, topped with reserved bacon.

Nutrition Per Serving: 84 calories, 1g total fat, 0g sat fat, 1mg cholesterol, 231mg sodium, 17g carbohydrate, 2 fiber, 3g protein

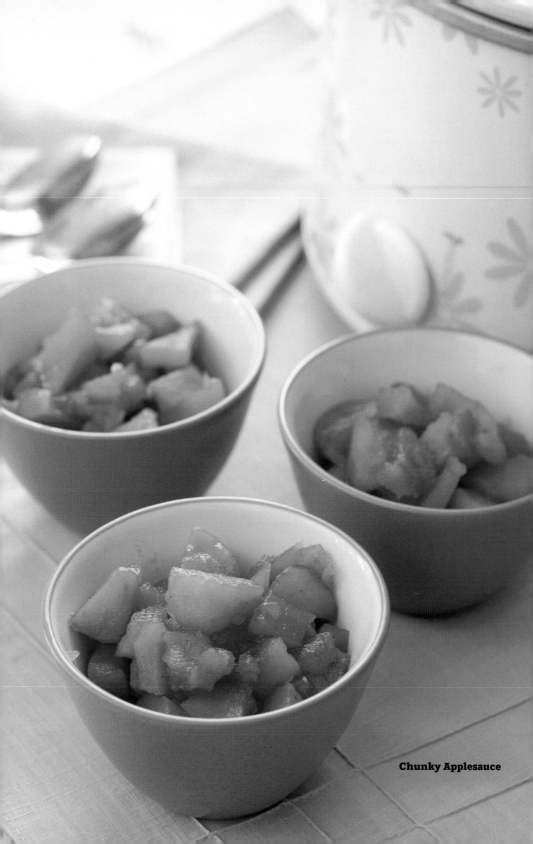

Chunky Applesauce

Lisa Hays, Crocker, MO

Garden-Style Fettuccine

What a delicious, nutritious meatless meal! It's packed full of veggies and yummy cheese...what more could you ask for?

Makes 12 servings

1 zucchini, sliced 1/4-inch thick
1 yellow squash, sliced 1/4-inch thick
2 carrots, peeled and thinly sliced
1-1/2 c. sliced mushrooms
10-oz. pkg. frozen broccoli cuts
4 green onions, sliced
1 clove garlic, minced
1/2 t. dried basil
1/4 t. salt
1/2 t. pepper
1 c. grated Parmesan cheese
12-oz. pkg. fettuccine pasta, cooked
1 c. shredded mozzarella cheese
1 c. 1% low-fat milk
2 egg yolks, beaten

Place vegetables, seasonings and Parmesan cheese in a slow cooker. Cover and cook on high setting for 2 hours. Add remaining ingredients to slow cooker; stir well. Reduce heat to low setting; cover and cook an additional 15 to 30 minutes.

Nutrition Per Serving: 180 calories, 6g total fat, 3g sat fat, 60mg cholesterol, 277mg sodium, 19g carbohydrate, 2g fiber, 10g protein

Patricia Wissler, Harrisburg, PA

Slow-Cooked Creamy Potatoes

So convenient for potlucks and holiday dinners.

Makes 8 servings

4 green onions, chopped
2 cloves garlic, minced
8 potatoes, sliced and divided
1/2 t. salt, divided
1/4 t. pepper, divided
8-oz. pkg. 1/3-less-fat cream cheese, diced and divided

Combine green onions and garlic in a small bowl; set aside. Layer 1/4 of the potato slices in a greased slow cooker; sprinkle with half of salt and pepper. Top with 1/3 each of cream cheese and green onion mixture. Repeat layers twice, ending with potatoes; sprinkle with salt and pepper. Cover and cook on high setting for 3 hours. Stir to blend melted cheese; cover and cook for an additional hour. Stir well and mash slightly before serving.

Nutrition Per Serving: 199 calories, 6g total fat, 3g sat fat, 20mg cholesterol, 352mg sodium, 29g carbohydrate, 2g fiber, 7g protein

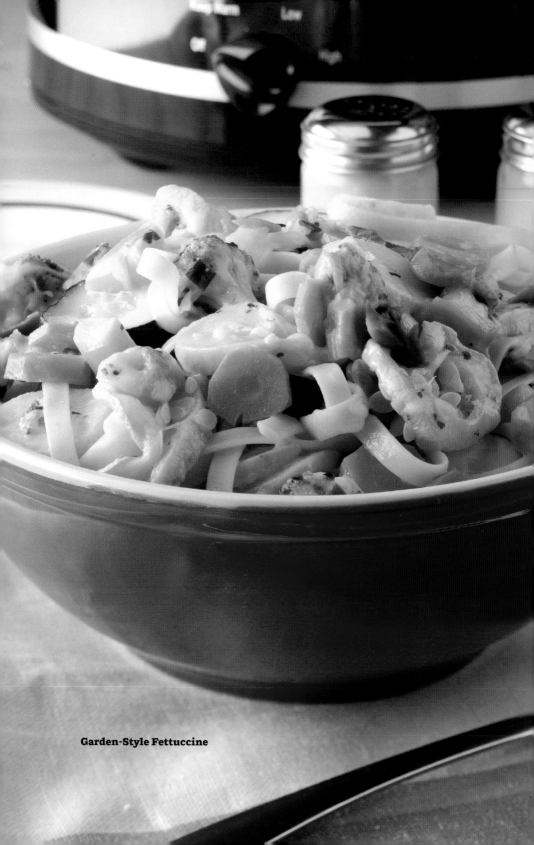

Garden-Style Fettuccine

Paula Schwenk, Pennsdale, PA

Slow-Cooker Mac & Cheese

So cheesy and satisfying...and it's a snap to put together.

Makes 14 servings

8-oz. pkg. elbow macaroni, cooked
1 T. olive oil
12-oz. can 2% reduced-fat evaporated milk
1-1/2 c. 2% reduced-fat milk
3 c. reduced-fat pasteurized process cheese spread, shredded
1/4 c. butter
2 T. dried, minced onion

Combine cooked macaroni and oil; toss to coat. Pour into a lightly greased slow cooker; stir in remaining ingredients. Cover and cook on low setting for 3 to 4 hours, stirring occasionally.

Nutrition Per Serving: 184 calories, 8g total fat, 4g sat fat, 25mg cholesterol, 450mg sodium, 18g carbohydrate, 1g fiber, 9g protein

★ SAVVY SWAP ★ Try penne pasta or small shell pasta for a simple variation.

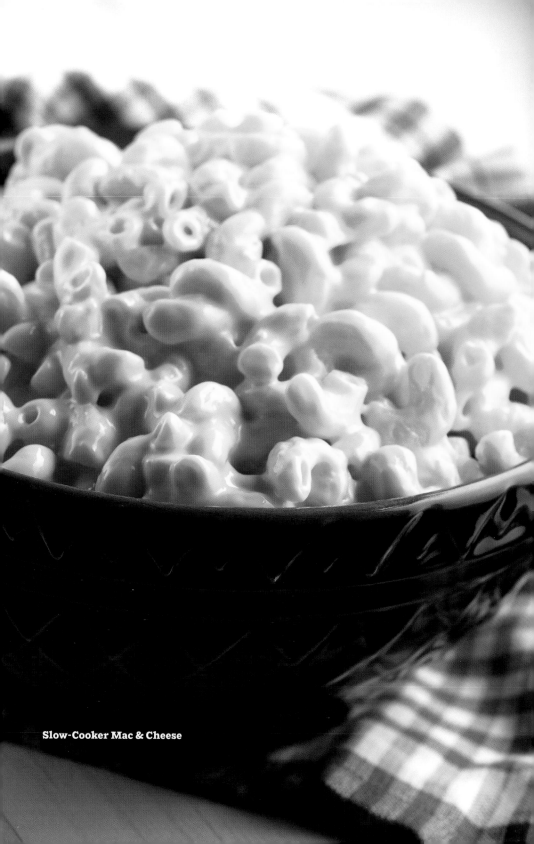

Slow-Cooker Mac & Cheese

Nancy Girard, Chesapeake, VA

Garlic Smashed Potatoes

This 5-ingredient side dish comes together right in your slow cooker, making for quick clean-up too.

Makes 8 servings

3 lbs. redskin potatoes, quartered
4 cloves garlic, minced
2 T. olive oil
1 t. salt
1/2 c. water
1/2 c. spreadable 1/3-less-fat cream
    cheese with chives and onions
1/4 to 1/2 c. 2% reduced-fat milk

Place potatoes in a slow cooker. Add garlic, oil, salt and water; mix well to coat potatoes. Cover and cook on high setting for 3-1/2 to 4-1/2 hours, until potatoes are tender. Mash potatoes with a potato masher or fork. Stir in cream cheese until well blended; add enough milk for a soft consistency. Serve immediately, or keep warm for up to 2 hours in slow cooker on low setting.

Nutrition Per Serving: 190 calories, 6g total fat, 2g sat fat, 4mg cholesterol, 411mg sodium, 28g carbohydrate, 3g fiber, 5g protein

★ SAVVY SWAP ★ For a milder flavor, use plain 1/3-less-fat cream cheese spread.

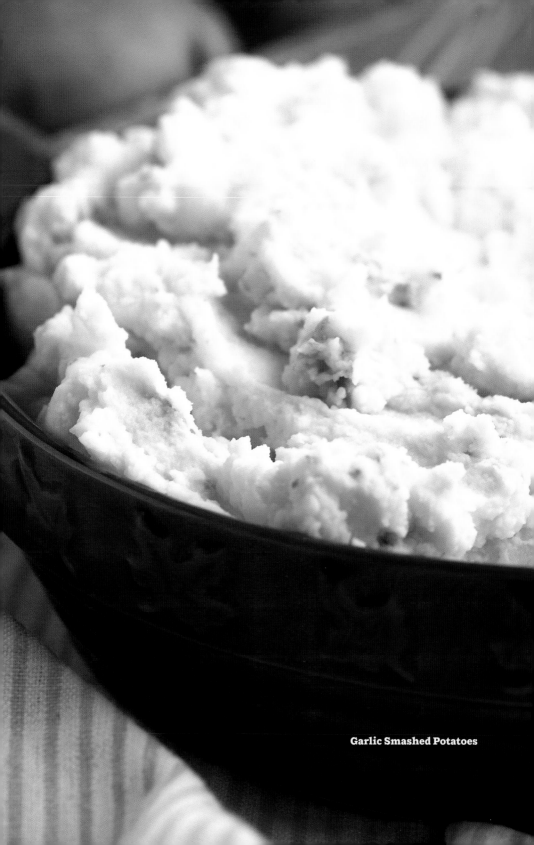

Garlic Smashed Potatoes

SIDES

Angela Murphy, Tempe AZ

Savory Spinach Soufflé

Try using Swiss cheese instead of Cheddar for something deliciously different.

Makes 12 servings

2 16-oz.pkgs. frozen chopped
  spinach, thawed and well drained
1/4 c. onion, grated
8-oz. pkg. 1/3-less-fat cream cheese,
  softened
1/2 c. reduced-fat mayonnaise
1/2 c. shredded reduced-fat Cheddar
  cheese
2 eggs, beaten
1/4 t. pepper
1/8 t. nutmeg

In a bowl, mix together spinach and onion; set aside. In a separate bowl, beat together remaining ingredients until well blended; fold into spinach mixture. Spoon into a lightly greased slow cooker. Cover and cook on high setting for 2 to 3 hours, until set.

Nutrition Per Serving: 122 calories, 9g total fat, 3g sat fat, 54mg cholesterol, 225mg sodium, 5g carbohydrate, 2g fiber, 7g protein

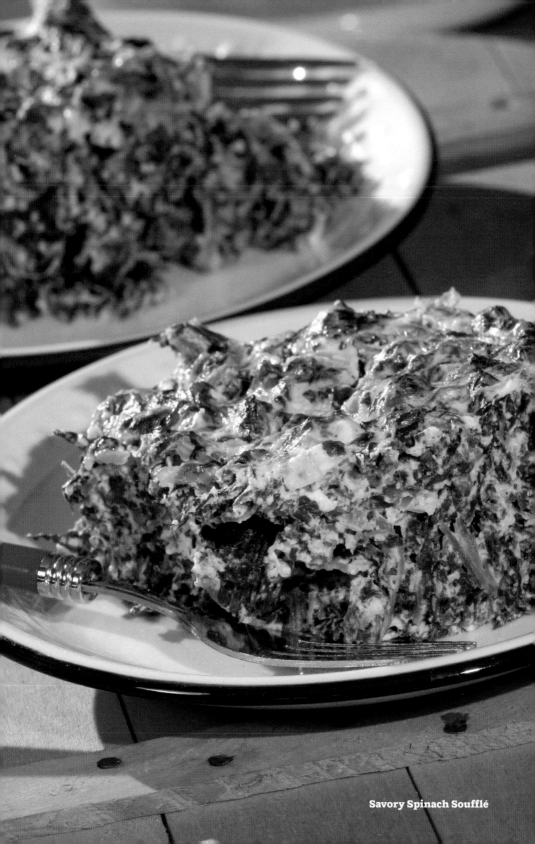

Savory Spinach Soufflé

Fawn McKenzie, Wenatchee, WA

Autumn Apple-Pecan Dressing

Made in the slow cooker, this side dish frees up your oven for a tasty roast chicken.

Makes 12 servings

4 c. soft bread cubes
1 c. saltine crackers, crushed
1-1/2 c. apples, peeled, cored and
    chopped
1 c. chopped pecans
1 c. onion, chopped
1 c. celery, chopped
2/3 c. low-sodium chicken broth
1/4 c. butter, melted
2 eggs, beaten
1/2 t. pepper
1/2 t. dried sage

Combine bread cubes, cracker crumbs, apples, pecans, onion and celery in a slow cooker; set aside. In a small bowl, mix remaining ingredients until well blended. Pour into slow cooker and toss to coat. Cover and cook on low setting for 4 to 5 hours, until dressing is puffed and golden around edges.

Nutrition Per Serving: 188 calories, 12g total fat, 4g sat fat, 46mg cholesterol, 181mg sodium, 17g carbohydrate, 2g fiber, 4g protein

★ SAVVY SWAP ★ You can use walnuts in place of the pecans, if you wish.

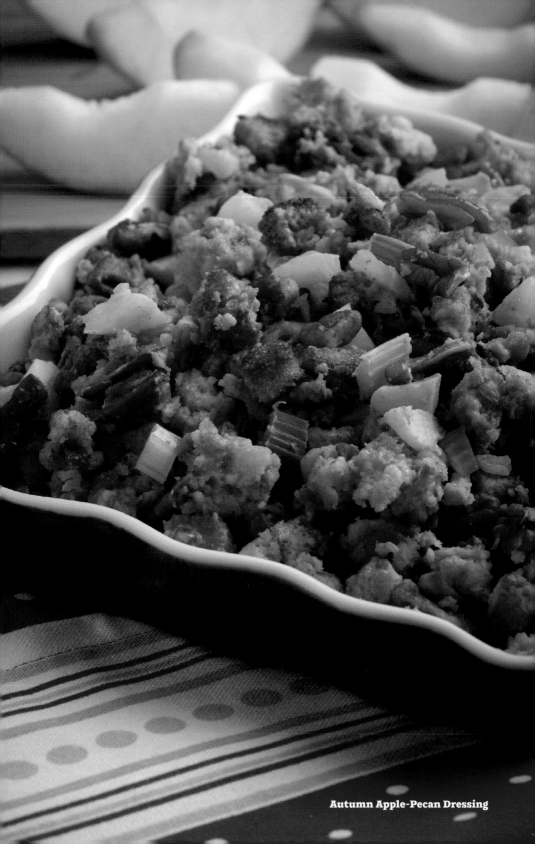

Autumn Apple-Pecan Dressing

Jo Ann, Gooseberry Patch

Spoon Bread Florentine

A deliciously different side that's so simple to make.

Makes 12 servings

10-oz. pkg. frozen chopped spinach,
   thawed and drained
6 green onions, sliced
1 red pepper, chopped
5-1/2 oz. pkg. cornbread mix
4 eggs, beaten
1/2 c. butter, melted
1 c. 1% low-fat cottage cheese
1-1/4 t. seasoned salt

Combine all ingredients in a large bowl; mix well. Spoon into a lightly greased slow cooker. Cover, with lid slightly ajar to allow moisture to escape. Cook on low setting for 3 to 4 hours, or on high setting for 1-3/4 to 2 hours, until edges are golden and a knife tip inserted in center tests clean.

Nutrition Per Serving: 162 calories, 10g total fat, 6g sat fat, 93mg cholesterol, 286mg sodium, 17g carbohydrate, 2g fiber, 7g protein

Annette Ingram, Grand Rapids, MI

Savory Corn Spoon Bread

Country-style flavor, so easy to fix.

Makes 8 servings

1 c. yellow cornmeal
2 t. baking powder
2 eggs, beaten
1 c. 1% low-fat buttermilk
2 T. oil
14-3/4 oz. can creamed corn
1 c. shredded reduced-fat sharp
   Cheddar cheese
Optional: 1 T. canned diced green
   chiles

In a bowl, beat together all ingredients. Pour batter into a greased 4-quart slow cooker. Cover and cook on low setting for 4 hours, or until a toothpick inserted in the center tests clean. Serve warm.

Nutrition Per Serving: 177 calories, 5g total fat, 3 sat fat, 66mg cholesterol, 309mg sodium, 23g carbohydrate, 1g fiber, 9g protein

★ SAVVY SWAP ★ Use frozen chopped kale in place of the spinach.

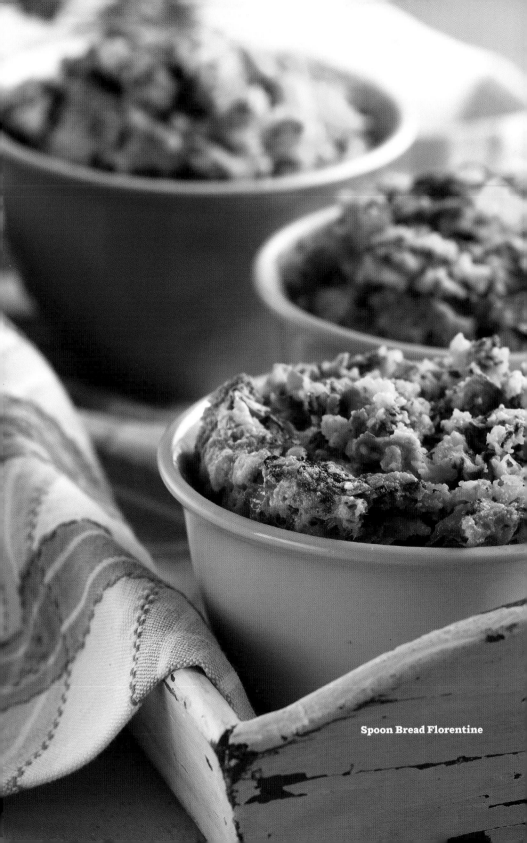

Spoon Bread Florentine

Debra Crisp, Grants Pass, OR

Cow-Country Beans

My family especially likes these yummy slow-cooker beans served over freshly made potato pancakes.

Makes 14 servings

3 c. dried red beans, rinsed and sorted
1 lb. cooked lean ham, cubed
1 onion, sliced
1 c. celery, diced
8-oz. can tomato sauce
2 T. bacon bits
2 T. chili powder
1 T. brown sugar
2 t. garlic powder
1/2 t. salt
1/2 t. smoke-flavored cooking sauce

Cover dried beans with water in a bowl; soak overnight. Drain beans; combine with remaining ingredients in a slow cooker. Cover and cook on high setting for 8 to 10 hours.

Nutrition Per Serving: 174 calories, 2g total fat, 1g sat fat, 15mg cholesterol, 591mg sodium, 24g carbohydrate, 7g fiber, 15g protein

★ SAVVY SWAP ★ Make this recipe with 2 slices cooked and crumbled center-cut bacon instead of bacon bits.

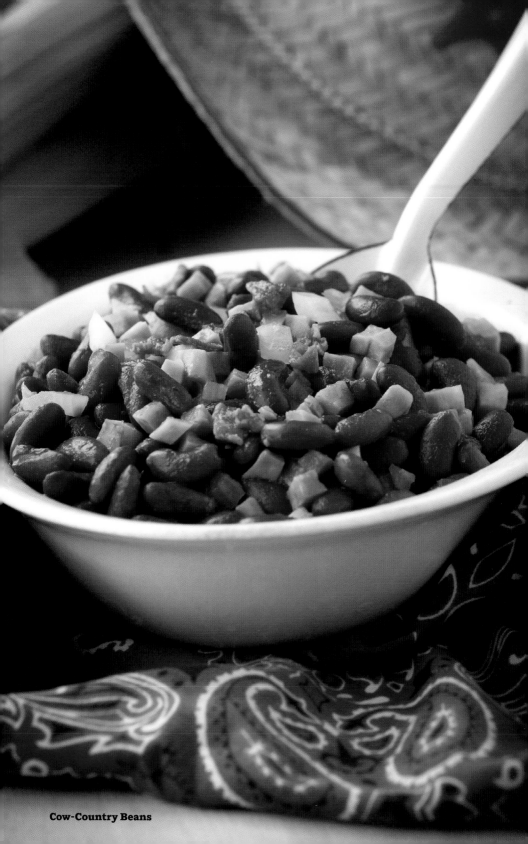

Cow-Country Beans

Beverley Williams, San Antonio, TX

Old-Fashioned Baked Beans

This was my grandmother's recipe. I grew up eating these beans in Tennessee. I usually do the first step overnight.

Makes 10 servings

2 c. dried Great Northern Beans, rinsed and sorted
5 c. water
1/2 c. onion, finely chopped
2 thick slices bacon, coarsely chopped
1-1/2 t. salt
2 T. brown sugar, packed
1/4 c. catsup
1 t. dry mustard
1/4 c. molasses

Place dried beans in a slow cooker. Add water, onion, bacon and salt. Cover and cook on high setting for 8 to 10 hours. Drain beans and return to slow cooker, reserving one cup of the liquid. Add remaining ingredients along with reserved liquid; mix well. Cover and cook on high setting for an addition one to 2 hours..

Nutrition Per Serving: 176 calories, 1g total fat, 0g sat fat, 1mg cholesterol, 455mg sodium, 34g carbohydrate, 8g fiber, 9g protein

Teresa Grimsley, Alamosa, CO

Beans Southwestern Style

I've developed this recipe over time, and it is absolutely the best bean recipe I've ever had! Make it a meal by doubling your serving size and pairing it with a salad.

Makes 14 servings

6 c. low-sodium chicken broth
1 onion, chopped
2 T. diced green chiles
1 carrot, peeled and chopped
1 stalk celery, chopped
14-1/2 oz. can diced tomatoes
4 cloves garlic, finely chopped
1 T. ground cumin
3 c. dried pinto beans
1 c. dried black beans
1-1/2 lb. pork shoulder roast, fat trimmed
Optional: chopped fresh cilantro, salsa verde, reduced-fat sour cream

Combine broth, vegetables, tomatoes with juice, garlic and cumin in a slow cooker. Add beans and pork to broth mixture. Cover and cook on low setting for 8 hours, until beans are tender and pork pulls apart easily. Remove pork from slow cooker and shred; set aside. Using a blender or immersion blender, purée about half of the bean and liquid mixture. Spoon pork back into slow cooker; mix well. Top servings with cilantro, salsa and sour cream, if desired.

Nutrition Per Serving: 207 calories, 1g total fat, 0g sat fat, 2mg cholesterol, 111mg sodium, 37g carbohydrate, 12g fiber, 14g protein

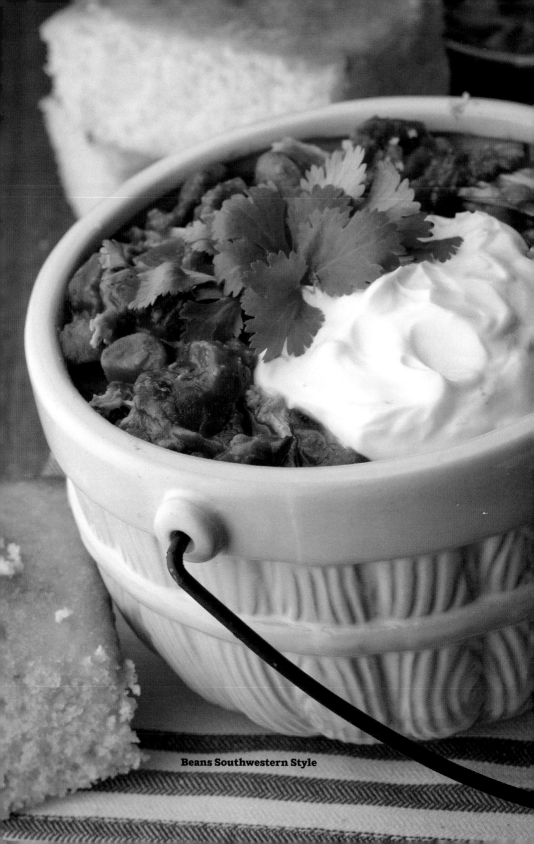

Beans Southwestern Style

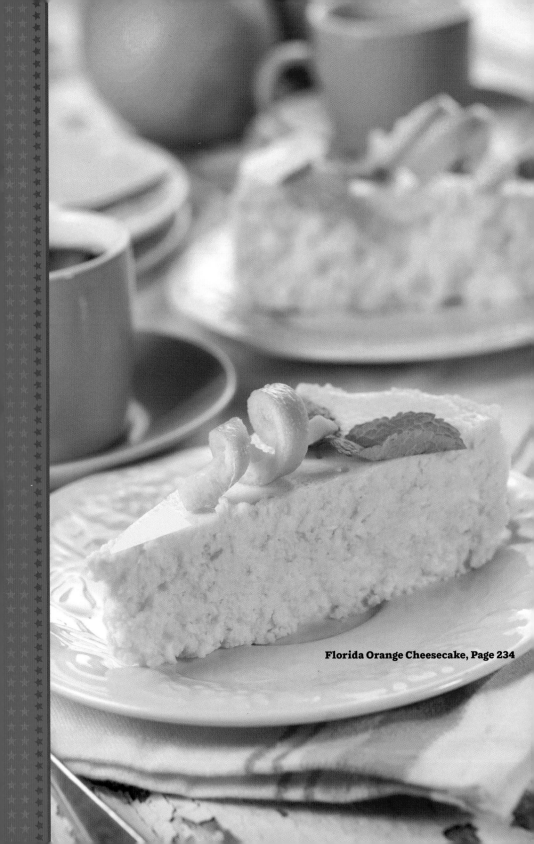

Florida Orange Cheesecake, Page 234

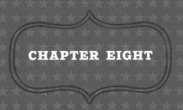

CHAPTER EIGHT

Snacks & Desserts

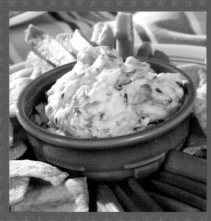

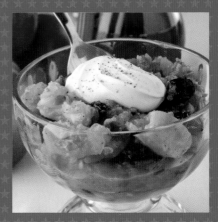

Spinach-Artichoke Dip, Page 222

Honeyed Apple Treat, Page 246

Marlene Darnell, Newport Beach, CA

Slow-Cooked Scrumptious Salsa

Nothing beats the taste of fresh, homemade salsa. This recipe is so simple, I make it all the time with fresh produce from my backyard garden. I give it as gifts and make sure to pass the recipe along with it!

Makes 8 servings

10 roma tomatoes, cored
2 cloves garlic
1 onion, cut into wedges
2 jalapeño peppers, seeded and chopped
1/4 c. fresh cilantro, coarsely chopped
1/2 t. salt

Combine tomatoes, garlic and onion in a slow cooker. Cover and cook on high setting for 2-1/2 to 3 hours, until vegetables are tender. Remove crock and let cool. Combine cooled tomato mixture and remaining ingredients in a food processor or blender. Process to desired consistency. May be refrigerated in a covered container for about one week.

Nutrition Per Serving: 21 calories, 8g total fat, 0g sat fat, 0mg cholesterol, 0mg sodium, 5g carbohydrate, 1g fiber, 1g protein

★ LOW-CAL ADD-ON ★ **Try this fresh salsa with multi-grain tortilla chips. A one-ounce serving has 150 calories.**

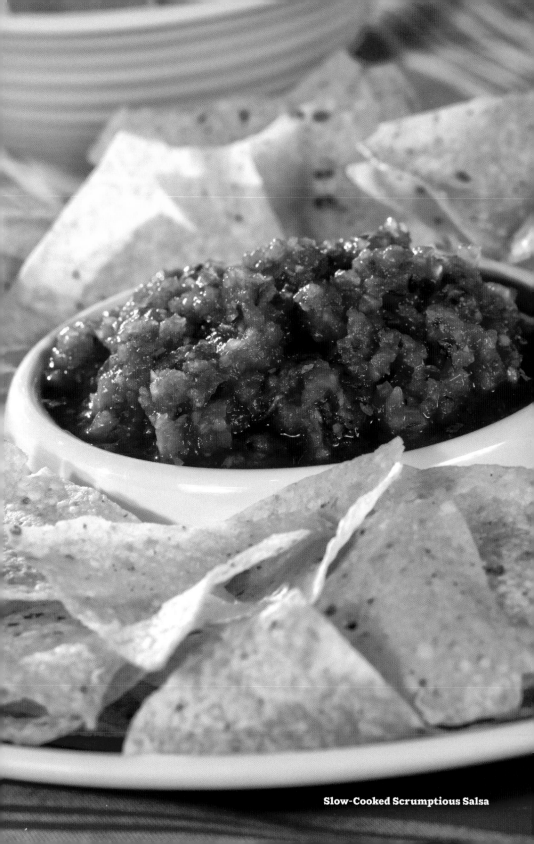

Slow-Cooked Scrumptious Salsa

Darcy Geiger, Columbia City, IN

South-of-the-Border Dip

I make this dip for get-togethers...
it's very easy and yummy!

Makes 24 servings

2 lbs. lean ground turkey sausage,
    browned and drained
3 14-1/2 oz. cans diced tomatoes with
    green chiles
1 c. favorite salsa
2 c. canned black beans, drained
2 c. canned corn, drained
8-oz. pkg. reduced-fat sharp Cheddar
    cheese or queso blanco pasteurized
    process cheese, cubed
8-oz. pkg. 1/3-less-fat cream cheese,
    cubed
2 9-oz. pkgs. multi-grain tortilla
    chips

Combine sausage, tomatoes with juice
and remaining ingredients except
tortilla chips in a slow cooker; mix
gently. Cover and cook on low setting
for about 4 hours, until cheeses are
melted. Stir before serving. Serve
warm with tortilla chips.

Nutrition Per Serving: 251 calories, 13g
total fat, 4g sat fat, 30mg cholesterol, 601
sodium, 22g carbohydrate, 4g fiber, 15g
protein

Vickie, Gooseberry Patch

Chipotle-Black Bean Dip

I am always asked to take this smoky,
spicy bean dip wherever I go...I've
even started bringing the recipe
to share.

Makes 12 servings

16-oz. can fat-free refried beans
15-oz. can black beans, drained and
    rinsed
11-oz. can sweet corn & diced peppers,
    drained
1 c. chunky salsa
2 chipotle chiles in adobo sauce,
    chopped and 2 t. adobo sauce reserved
1-1/2 c. shredded reduced-fat Cheddar
    cheese, divided
4 green onions, chopped
9-oz. pkg. multi-grain tortilla chips

Mix together beans, corn, salsa, chiles,
reserved adobo sauce and one cup
cheese in a slow cooker. Cover and cook
on low setting for 3 to 4 hours, stirring
after 2 hours. Sprinkle with remaining
cheese and onions. Keep warm on low
setting; serve with tortilla chips.

Nutrition Per Serving: 221 calories, 9g total
fat, 3g sat fat, 11mg cholesterol, 650mg
sodium, 26g carbohydrate, 6g fiber, 9g protein

★ SAVVY SWAP ★ Serve with baguette toasts
or pita chips instead of tortilla chips for variety.

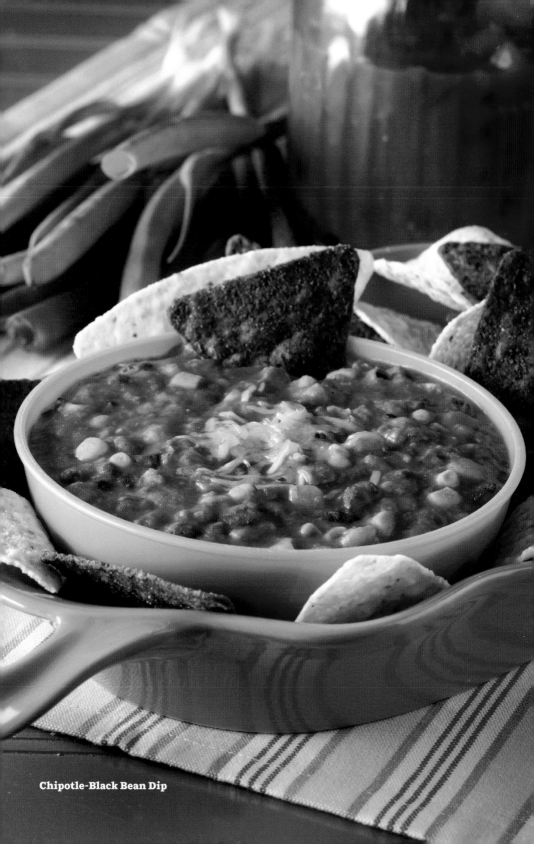

Chipotle-Black Bean Dip

Lori Steen, Aloha, OR

Cheddar Fondue

This ooey-gooey dip is an all-time favorite in our house! We make it during football season and the holidays when we have guests over.

Makes 16 servings

1/4 c. butter
1/4 c. all-purpose flour
1/2 t. salt
1/2 t. pepper
1/4 t. Worcestershire sauce
1/4 t. dry mustard
1-1/2 c. 2% reduced-fat milk
8-oz. pkg. shredded reduced-fat
  Cheddar cheese
16-oz. loaf French bread, cubed

Melt butter in a saucepan over medium heat. Whisk in flour, salt, pepper, Worcestershire sauce and mustard until smooth. Gradually add milk; boil for 2 minutes or until thickened, whisking constantly. Reduce heat; add cheese, stirring until melted. Transfer to a mini slow cooker set on low and keep warm. Serve with bread cubes for dipping.

Nutrition Per Serving: 167 calories, 7g total fat, 4g sat fat, 21mg cholesterol, 372mg sodium, 17g carbohydrate, 1g fiber, 9g protein

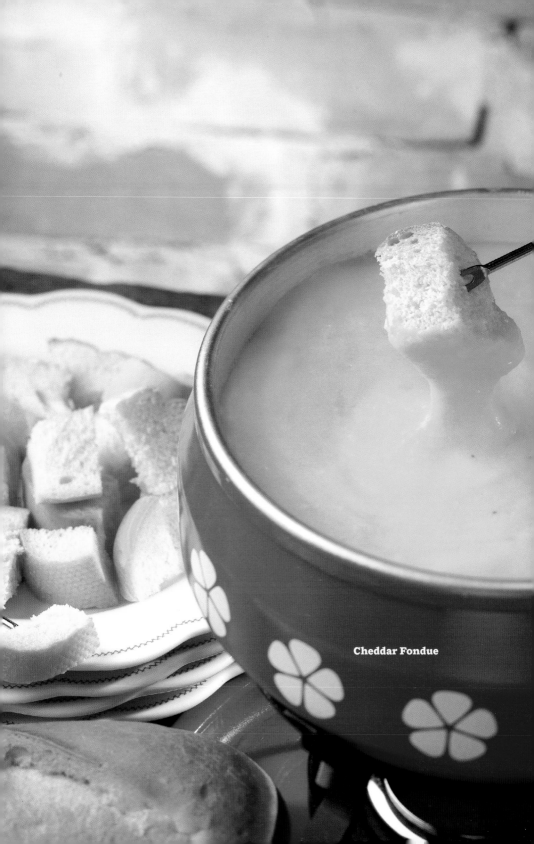

Cheddar Fondue

Vickie, Gooseberry Patch

Hot Buffalo Dip

This spicy dip features 3 cheeses and is fit for any party. One of my favorite dips...oh-so easy to make and we all love it!

Makes 16 servings

4 6-oz. boneless, skinless chicken breasts, cooked and chopped
2 8-oz. pkgs. 1/3-less-fat cream cheese, cubed and softened
1 c. hot wing sauce
1/2 c. shredded reduced-fat Cheddar cheese
1/4 c. light blue cheese salad dressing

In a slow cooker, mix together all ingredients. Cover and cook on low setting for 3 to 4 hours.

Nutrition Per Serving: 141 calories, 9g total fat, 4g sat fat, 55mg cholesterol, 526mg sodium, 2g carbohydrate, 0g fiber, 14g protein

Tiffany Brinkley, Broomfield, CO

Zesty Cider-Cheddar Dip

My family just loves cheese! We're always trying new recipes for hot cheese dip and fondue. So when I found this recipe with an added zip of cider, we were pretty excited. We love it...you will too!

Makes 16 servings

1 T. all-purpose flour
1 t. dry mustard
1/2 c. hard cider or apple cider
1 t. Worcestershire sauce
1 t. hot pepper sauce
2 c. shredded reduced-fat Cheddar cheese
1/2 lb. reduced-fat pasteurized process cheese, cubed

Add flour and mustard to a 2-quart slow cooker; mix well and set aside. In a cup, combine cider and sauces; add to flour mixture and mix well. Stir in cheese. Cover and cook on high setting for 1-1/2 hours, stirring twice, until cheese is melted and smooth.

Nutrition Per Serving: 77 calories, 5g total fat, 3g sat fat, 16mg cholesterol, 356mg sodium, 3g carbohydrate, 0g fiber, 6g protein

★ LOW-CAL ADD-ON ★ Apple slices and pretzel sticks make the best dippers for this appetizer. A one-cup serving of sliced apples and a 1/2-ounce serving of pretzels each contain only about 50 calories.

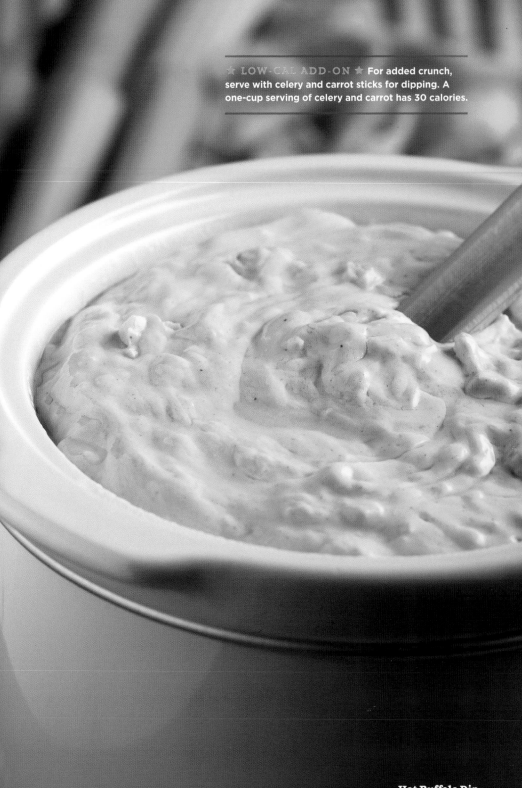

★ LOW-CAL ADD-ON ★ For added crunch, serve with celery and carrot sticks for dipping. A one-cup serving of celery and carrot has 30 calories.

Hot Buffalo Dip

Rachel Adams, Fort Lewis, WA

Spinach-Artichoke Dip

Serve with pita chips and sliced vegetables for dipping.

Makes 16 servings

14-oz. can artichoke hearts, drained
  and chopped
2 bunches fresh spinach, chopped
2 8-oz. pkgs. 1/3-less-fat cream
  cheese, softened and cubed
2-1/2 c. shredded Monterey Jack
  cheese
2-1/2 c. shredded part-skim
  mozzarella cheese
3 cloves garlic, minced
1/4 t. pepper

Combine chopped artichokes, spinach and cheeses in a slow cooker; mix well. Stir in garlic and pepper. Cover and cook on high setting for about one to 2 hours, stirring occasionally, until cheeses are melted and dip is smooth. Reduce heat to low setting to keep warm.

Nutrition Per Serving: 204 calories, 1g total fat, 16g sat fat, 49mg cholesterol, 382mg sodium, 5g carbohydrate, 1g fiber, 13g protein

Janice Dorsey, San Antonio, TX

Glazed Kielbasa Bites

Everybody loves these savory morsels of sausage from the slow cooker!

Makes 16 servings

1 lb. turkey Kielbasa sausage,
  cut into bite-size slices
1 c. apricot preserves
1/2 c. maple syrup
2 T. bourbon or maple syrup

Combine all ingredients in a slow cooker; cover and cook on low setting for 4 hours.

Nutrition Per Serving: 123 calories, 2g total fat, 1g sat fat, 16mg cholesterol, 231mg sodium, 21g carbohydrate, 1g fiber, 5g protein

---

★ SAVVY SWAP ★ Pineapple or peach preserves would be a delicious sub for the apricot preserves in this easy appetizer.

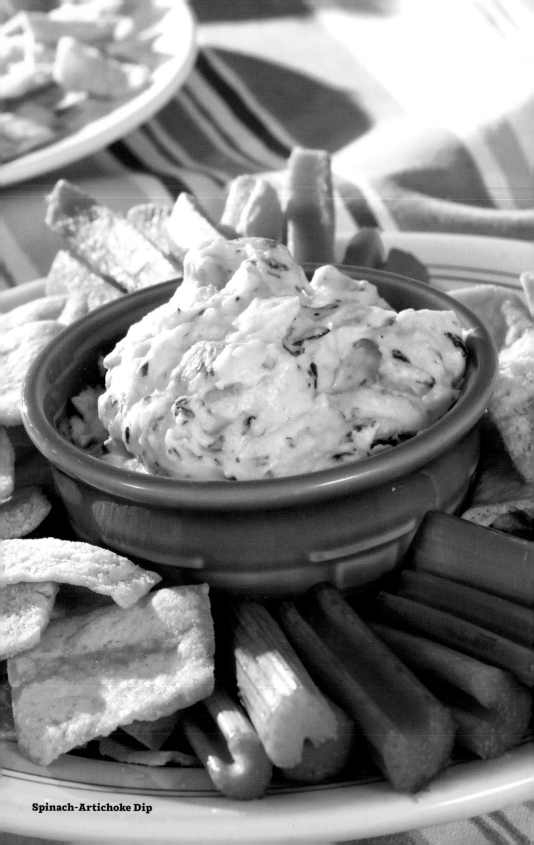

Spinach-Artichoke Dip

Kathy Grashoff, Fort Wayne, IN

Bacon-Horseradish Dip

Put a slow cooker to work cooking up this creamy, cheesy dip...it's out of this world!

Makes 24 servings

3 8-oz. pkgs. 1/3-less-fat cream
   cheese, softened
12-oz. pkg. shredded reduced-fat
   Cheddar cheese
1 c. half-and-half
1/3 c. green onion, chopped
3 cloves garlic, minced
3 T. prepared horseradish
1 T. Worcestershire sauce
1/2 t. pepper
12 slices center-cut bacon, crisply
   cooked and crumbled

Combine all ingredients except bacon in a slow cooker. Cover and cook on low setting for 4 to 5 hours, or on high setting for 2 to 2-1/2 hours, stirring once halfway through. Just before serving, stir in bacon.

Nutrition Per Serving: 218 calories, 17g total fat, 10g sat fat, 55mg cholesterol, 393mg sodium, 3g carbohydrate, 0g fiber, 13g protein

Shannon Finewood, Corpus Cristi, TX

Pizza Fondue

All the tasty flavors of pizza are mixed up together in one crowd-pleasing appetizer. Serve with Italian bread cubes, pepperoni chunks, whole mushrooms or green pepper slices.

Makes 16 servings

28-oz. jar spaghetti sauce
16-oz. pkg. shredded part-skim
   mozzarella cheese
1/4 c. grated Parmesan cheese
2 T. dried oregano
2 T. dried parsley
1 T. garlic powder
1 t. dried, minced onion

Combine sauce, cheeses and seasonings in a slow cooker; mix well. Cover and cook on low setting for 2 hours, or until warmed through and cheese is melted. Stir before serving.

Nutrition Per Serving: 111 calories, 7g total fat, 4g sat fat, 22mg cholesterol, 411mg sodium, 5g carbohydrate, 1g fiber, 8g protein

★ LOW-CAL ADD-ON ★ Try cubes of crusty Italian bread, sourdough or even tiny boiled new potatoes with this dreamy fondue. A 1/2-cup serving of each dipper has less than 100 calories.

★ LOW-CAL ADD-ON ★ Serve with bagel chips. Fifteen chips have 130 calories.

Bacon-Horseradish Dip

Connie Fortune, Covington, OH

Sugared Walnuts

A fix & forget version of this holiday favorite. It's also a filling snack to keep on hand during the rest of the year.

Makes 16 servings

1 lb. walnut halves
1/2 c. butter, melted
1/2 c. powdered sugar
1-1/2 t. cinnamon
1/4 t. ground cloves
1/4 t. ground ginger

Preheat a slow cooker on high setting for 15 minutes. Add walnuts and butter, stirring to mix well. Add powdered sugar; mix until coated evenly. Cover and cook on high setting for 15 minutes. Reduce heat to low setting. Cook, uncovered, stirring occasionally, for 2 to 3 hours, or until nuts are coated with a crisp glaze. Transfer nuts to a serving bowl. Combine spices in a small bowl and sprinkle over nuts, stirring to coat evenly. Cool before serving. Store in an airtight container.

Nutrition Per Serving: 251 calories, 24g total fat, 5g sat fat, 15mg cholesterol, 46mg sodium, 8g carbohydrate, 2g fiber, 4g protein

★ SAVVY SWAP ★ Pecans and almonds would make a nice alternative to the walnuts.

Jo Ann, Gooseberry Patch

Rosemary-White Bean Dip

Serve with assorted dippers such as crackers, toasted baguette slices and cherry tomatoes.

Makes 8 servings

3/4 c. dried white beans, rinsed and sorted
4 cloves garlic, minced
1 T. fresh rosemary, chopped
1 t. red pepper flakes
2 c. low-sodium vegetable broth
1 t. salt
7 T. olive oil
1-1/2 T. lemon juice
1 T. fresh parsley, chopped

Combine beans, garlic, rosemary, pepper flakes and broth in a slow cooker. Cover and cook on high setting for 3 hours, or until beans are soft and liquid is mostly absorbed. Remove crock and cool. Place cooled bean mixture into a blender; stir in oil and lemon juice. Process until dip reaches desired consistency. Spoon dip into a serving bowl; sprinkle with parsley.

Nutrition Per Serving: 175 calories, 12g total fat, 2g sat fat, 0mg cholesterol, 334mg sodium, 13g carbohydrate, 3g fiber, 5g protein

Christi Assink, South Haven, MI

Chocolate Peanut Clusters

A tasty sweet treat to keep on hand for an occasional snack or for gifting during the holiday season.

Makes 56 servings

2 16-oz. jars salted dry-roasted peanuts
32-oz. pkg. white melting chocolate, chopped
12-oz. pkg. semi-sweet chocolate chips
4-oz. pkg. sweet baking chocolate, chopped

Combine all ingredients in a slow cooker. Cover and cook on low setting for 1-1/2 hours. Turn off slow cooker. Let stand 20 minutes; stir until blended. Drop by rounded tablespoonsfuls onto wax paper. Let stand one hour, or until firm. Store clusters in airtight container, or freeze for up to one month.

Nutrition Per Serving: 220 calories, 15g total fat, 6g sat fat, 0mg cholesterol, 53mg sodium, 9g carbohydrate, 2g fiber, 6g protein

★ SKINNY SECRET ★ Make small clusters to keep the portion size of these sweet treats in check.

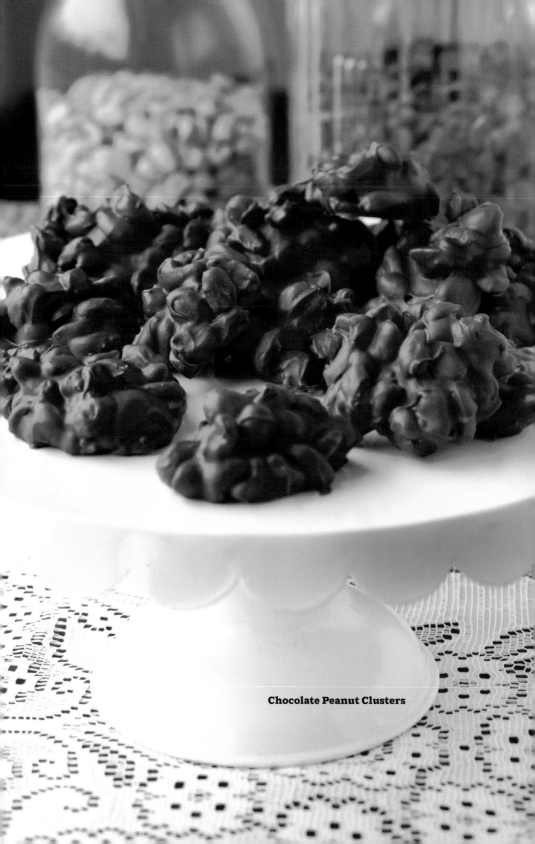

Chocolate Peanut Clusters

Becky Butler, Keller, TX

Roasted Cajun Pecans

When pecans start falling from their trees in September and October, it's the perfect time to roast them for snacking!

Makes 16 servings

1 t. chili powder
1 t. dried basil
1 t. dried oregano
1 t. dried thyme
1 t. salt
1/2 t. onion powder
1/2 t. garlic powder
1/4 t. cayenne pepper
1/4 c. butter, melted
1 lb. pecan halves

In a small bowl, mix together spices; set aside. Pour melted butter into a slow cooker; stir in pecans until evenly coated. Sprinkle spice mixture over pecans, stirring constantly, until evenly seasoned. Cover and cook on high setting for 12 to 15 minutes, stirring once. Remove lid from slow cooker and reduce heat to low setting. Cook, uncovered, for 2 hours, stirring occasionally. Remove pecans from slow cooker; cool on a paper towel-lined wire rack. Store in an airtight container.

Nutrition Per Serving: 221 calories, 23g total fat, 4g sat fat, 8mg cholesterol, 170mg sodium, 4g carbohydrate, 3g fiber, 3g protein

Carol Davis, Edmond, OK

Spice-Coated Pecans

We have an abundance of fresh pecans from our trees and this is such a great gift item. Sometimes I'll coat the finished clusters in melting chocolate...yummy!

Makes 16 servings

1 egg white, beaten
1 t. water
1/4 c. brown sugar, packed
1/4 c. sugar
1 t. cinnamon
1/4 t. nutmeg
1/4 t. allspice
4 c. pecan halves

Spray a 4-quart slow cooker with non-stick vegetable spray; set aside. In a large bowl, beat together egg white and water well. Stir in sugars and spices. Add pecans; turn to coat well and spoon into slow cooker. Cover and cook on low setting for 4 to 4-1/2 hours, stirring once after 2 hours. Spread pecans on non-stick aluminum foil; cool and break into clusters. Store in an airtight container.

Nutrition Per Serving: 197 calories, 18g total fat, 2g sat fat, 0mg cholesterol, 4mg sodium, 10g carbohydrate, 2g fiber, 3g protein

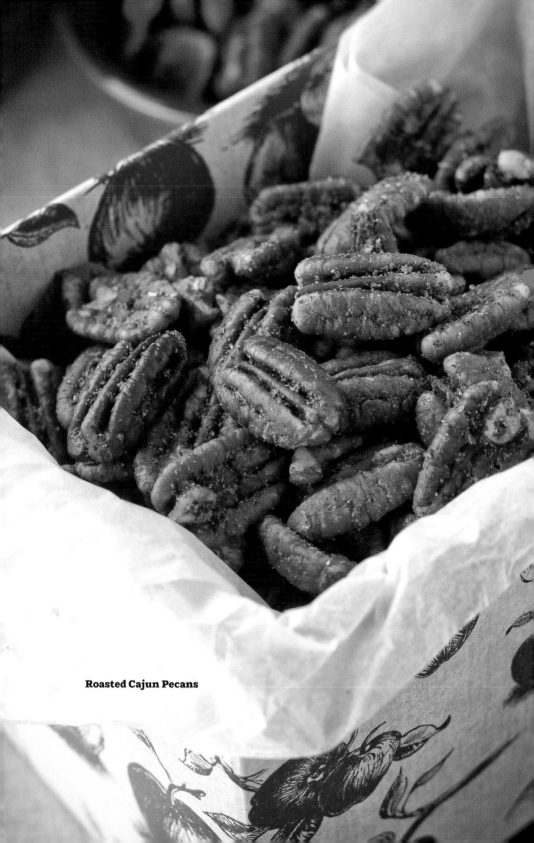

Roasted Cajun Pecans

Michelle Riihl, Windom, MN

Toffee Fondue

Use espresso or dark roast coffee for this recipe. The darker the coffee you use, the richer the flavor of the fondue.

Makes 14 servings

14-oz. pkg. caramels, unwrapped
1/4 c. 2% reduced-fat milk
1/4 c. strong black coffee
1/2 c. milk chocolate chips

Mix together caramels, milk, coffee and chocolate chips in a small slow cooker. Cover and cook on low setting until melted, about 2 to 3 hours. Stir well before serving.

Nutrition Per Serving: 143 calories, 4g total fat, 2g sat fat, 4mg cholesterol, 76mg sodium, 26g carbohydrate, 0g fiber, 2g protein

★ LOW-CAL ADD-ON ★ Apple wedges, banana chunks, marshmallows and angel food cake cubes make delightful dippers for fondue and have less than 100 calories per one-cup serving.

Janis Parr, Ontario, Canada

Tapioca Salad Dessert

This luscious dessert is rich and creamy...perfect for those times when you want to treat your family to something special. It's always a hit with everyone.

Makes 12 servings

2/3 c. large pearl tapioca, uncooked
1/2 c. sugar
1/8 t. salt
4 c. water
1 c. seedless grapes, halved
1 c. crushed pineapple, drained
11-oz. can mandarin oranges, drained
1 c. whipped cream

Mix together tapioca, sugar, salt and water in a 3-quart slow cooker. Cover and cook on high setting for 3 hours, or until tapioca pearls are almost transparent. Cool thoroughly in refrigerator. Just before serving, stir in fruit and whipped cream. Serve chilled.

Nutrition Per Serving: 119 calories, 3g total fat, 2g sat fat, 11mg cholesterol, 29mg sodium, 26 carbohydrate, 0g fiber, 0g protein

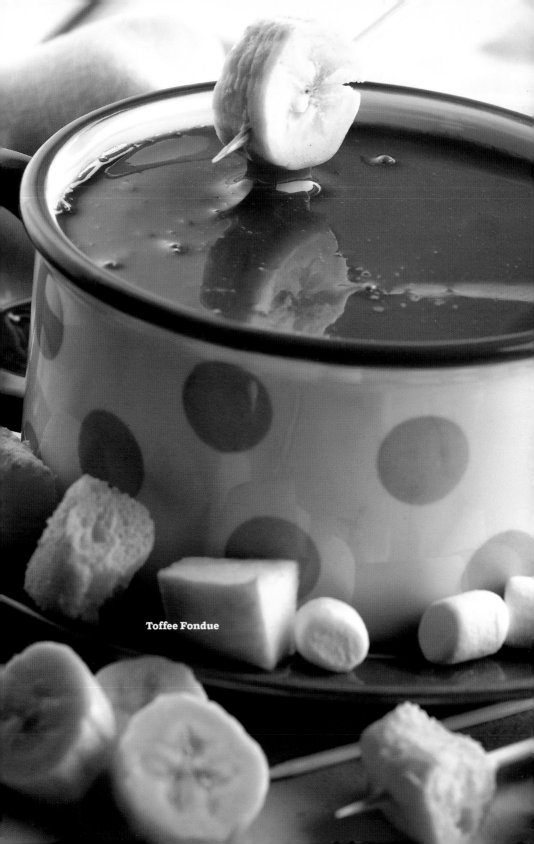

Toffee Fondue

Dana Cunningham, Lafayette, PA

Florida Orange Cheesecake

A citrusy cheesecake...I can't get enough of its unique flavor! Tastes amazing with a hot mug of coffee.

Makes 8 servings

1-1/2 c. 1/3-less-fat cream cheese, softened
1 T. all-purpose flour
1/2 c. sugar
2 T. orange juice
1/2 t. vanilla extract
3 eggs, lightly beaten
1/2 c. non-fat sour cream
1 t. orange zest
1 c. warm water
Optional: orange zest curls

In a large bowl, combine cream cheese, flour, sugar, juice and vanilla. Beat mixture with an electric mixer on medium speed until combined; beat in eggs until smooth. Mix in sour cream until smooth; stir in zest. Spoon filling into a lightly greased 1-1/2 quart casserole dish; cover tightly with aluminum foil. Pour warm water into a large slow cooker; set casserole dish in water. Cover and cook on high setting for 2-1/2 hours, or until center of cheesecake is set. Carefully remove casserole dish to a wire rack; uncover and cool cheesecake. When cool, cover and refrigerate for 4 hours. Garnish slices with curls of orange zest, if desired.

Nutrition Per Serving: 204 calories, 11g total fat, 6g sat fat, 113mg cholesterol, 179mg sodium, 17g carbohydrate, 0 fiber, 7g protein

★ SAVVY SWAP ★ Sub lemon or lime juice for the orange juice for a different citrus flavor.

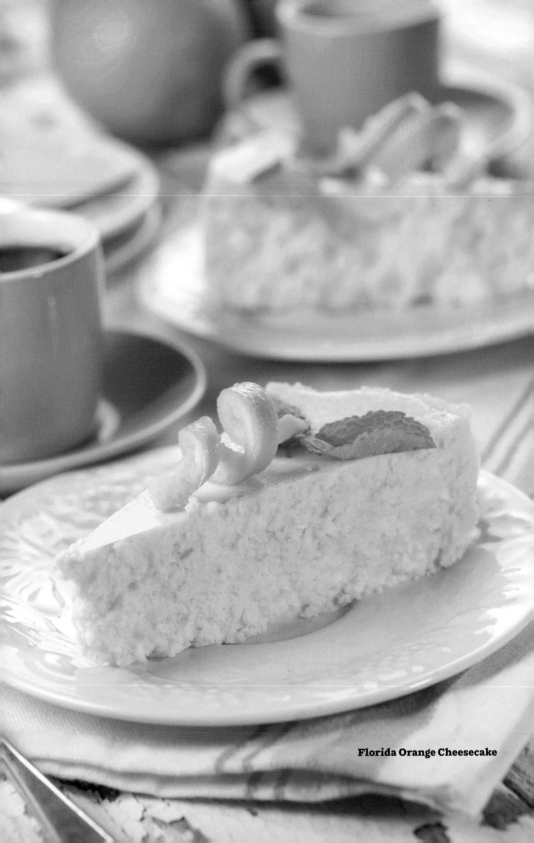

Florida Orange Cheesecake

Rochelle Rootes, Saint Francis, MN

Grandma's Apple Pie in a Crock

I remember the aroma that came from my grandma's kitchen every fall when she made this scrumptious dessert.

Makes 10 servings

8 tart apples, peeled, cored and sliced
3/4 c. milk
1/3 c. brown sugar, packed
1-1/4 t. cinnamon
2 eggs, beaten
1/4 t. allspice
1 t. vanilla extract
1/4 t. nutmeg
1 c. low-fat biscuit baking mix
3 T. cold butter, sliced

Spray a slow cooker with non-stick vegetable cooking spray. Layer all ingredients in the order listed. Cover and cook on low setting for 6 to 8 hours, until apples are tender and top is golden. Serve warm.

Nutrition Per Serving: 200 calories, 6g total fat, 3g sat fat, 54mg cholesterol, 156mg sodium, 37g carbohydrate, 4 fiber, 3g protein

---

★ SAVVY SWAP ★ **Try this treat with fresh peaches during the summer months when they're in season.**

Gretchen Hickman, Galva, IL

Crockery Apple Pie

I received this recipe from my great-aunt who owned an orchard. This smells heavenly when it's cooking, and it's perfect with served with a scoop of light vanilla bean ice cream.

Makes 12 servings

8 tart apples, peeled, cored and sliced
2 t. cinnamon
1/4 t. allspice
1/4 t. nutmeg
3/4 c. 2% reduced-fat milk
2 T. butter, softened
3/4 c. sugar
2 eggs, beaten
1 t. vanilla extract
1-1/2 c. low-fat biscuit baking mix, divided
1/3 c. brown sugar, packed
3 T. chilled butter

In a large bowl, toss apples with spices. Spoon apple mixture into a lightly greased slow cooker. In separate bowl, combine milk, softened butter, sugar, eggs, vanilla and 1/2 cup baking mix; stir until well mixed. Spoon batter over apples. Place remaining baking mix and brown sugar in small bowl. Cut in chilled butter until coarse crumbs form. Sprinkle over batter in slow cooker. Cover and cook on low setting for 6 to 7 hours.

Nutrition Per Serving: 253 calories, 7g total fat, 4g sat fat, 50mg cholesterol, 188mg sodium, 46g carbohydrate, 3g fiber, 3g protein

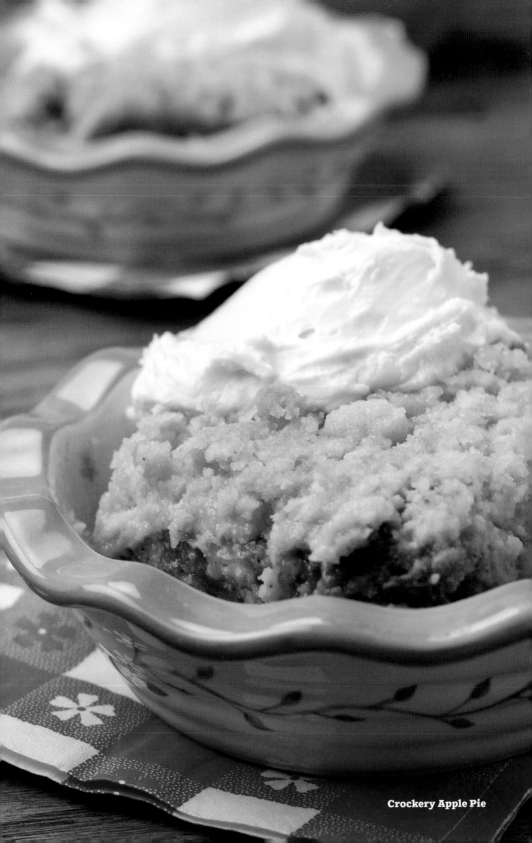

Crockery Apple Pie

Sandra Sullivan, Aurora, CO

Perfect Pumpkin-Apple Cake

No oven needed...so easy to do on the run! This tasty cake is perfect for when your oven is all tied up with other dishes.

Makes 24 servings

1/2 c. butter, softened
1-1/2 c. brown sugar, packed
1 c. canned pumpkin
3 eggs
2 c. all-purpose flour
2 t. baking powder
1 t. cinnamon
1/4 t. salt
Optional: chopped walnuts or pecans
21-oz. can apple pie filling
12-oz. container frozen whipped topping, thawed

In a large bowl, beat together butter and brown sugar with an electric mixer on low speed until well mixed. Beat in pumpkin and eggs until blended. In a separate bowl, sift together flour, baking powder, baking soda, cinnamon and salt. Slowly add flour mixture to butter mixture; beat for 2 minutes. Fold in nuts, if using. Spoon pie filling into a slow cooker. Cover and cook on high setting for 1-1/2 to 2 hours, until a toothpick tests clean. Garnish servings with a dollop of whipped topping.

Nutrition Per Serving: 208 calories, 8g total fat, 6g sat fat, 37mg cholesterol, 83mg sodium, 32g carbohydrate, 1 fiber, 2g protein

★ LOW-CAL ADD-ON ★ Sprinkle 2 teaspoons chopped nuts over each serving for a nice crunch and just 30 more calories.

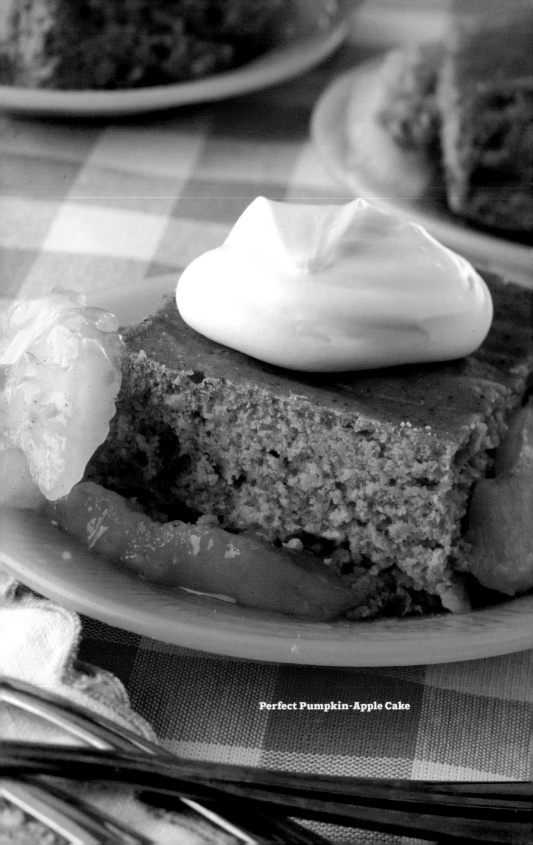

Perfect Pumpkin-Apple Cake

Sue Morrison, Blue Spring, MO

Ritzy Fruit Cobbler

This is an original recipe of mine. It's a very good way to use up odds & ends of frozen fruit.

Makes 8 servings

4 c. frozen blueberries, cherries,
   blackberries, strawberries,
   raspberries, sliced peaches or a
   mixture, divided
1 c. sugar, divided
1 sleeve reduced-fat round buttery
   crackers, divided
2 T. butter, softened
Optional: cinnamon to taste
juice of 1 lemon

Spray a slow cooker with non-stick vegetable spray. Add one cup frozen fruit; sprinkle with 1/4 cup sugar. Arrange 8 whole crackers on top. Continue layering, making 3 more layers of fruit, sugar and crackers. For top layer, crush remaining crackers; mix with butter and remaining sugar. Sprinkle cracker mixture on top; add cinnamon, if desired. Sprinkle with lemon juice. Cover and cook on low setting for one to 1-1/2 hours, until bubbly and fruit is juicy. Stir gently, breaking up crackers; the crackers will thicken the mixture.

Nutrition Per Serving: 188 calories, 3g total fat, 1g sat fat, 4mg cholesterol, 33mg sodium, 41g carbohydrate, 2g fiber, 1g protein

---

★ LOW-CAL ADD-ON ★ **Serve warm from slow cooker, topped with a 1/4-cup scoop of light vanilla ice cream for an additional 50 calories per serving.**

Chantel Bitter, Larose, LA

Coconut Rice Pudding

Garnish this creamy pudding with a sprinkle of pistachio nuts.

Makes 8 servings

1 c. medium-grain long-cooking rice, uncooked
1/2 t. salt
2 14-oz. cans light coconut milk
2-1/2 c. water
2/3 c. sugar
1-1/2 t. vanilla extract
1/2 t. garam masala or nutmeg

Spray a slow cooker with non-stick vegetable spray. Add uncooked rice and salt; set aside. Combine coconut milk, water and sugar in a saucepan; bring to a boil over medium heat. Add to slow cooker; stir well. Cover and cook on high setting for about 2 hours, until rice is tender. Stir in vanilla and spice. If pudding is too thin, stir gently until excess liquid is absorbed. If too dry, stir in a little hot water. Serve warm or chilled.

Nutrition Per Serving: 216 calories, 5g total fat, 4g sat fat, 0mg cholesterol, 181mg sodium, 41g carbohydrate, 1g fiber, 2g protein

Kathe Nych, Mercer, PA

Pumpkin Bread Pudding

Especially good in the autumn and at Thanksgiving...it fills the house with such a delicious pumpkin aroma! It's even great for breakfast. A terrific way to use up stale or leftover bread.

Makes 8 servings

3 c. bread, cubed
1/4 c. butter, melted
29-oz. can pumpkin
2 c. 2% reduced-fat milk
4 eggs, beaten
1/4 c. sugar
1 t. vanilla extract
1 t. cinnamon
1 t. nutmeg

Coat the inside of a slow cooker with non-stick vegetable spray. Combine bread and melted butter in a bowl; toss to coat. Add enough bread cubes to line slow cooker; set aside. In a separate bowl, beat together remaining ingredients; pour over bread cubes. Cover and cook on high setting for one hour, or on low setting for 3 to 4 hours.

Nutrition Per Serving: 221 calories, 10g total fat, 5g sat fat, 113mg cholesterol, xmg sodium, 24g carbohydrate, 3g fiber, 7g protein

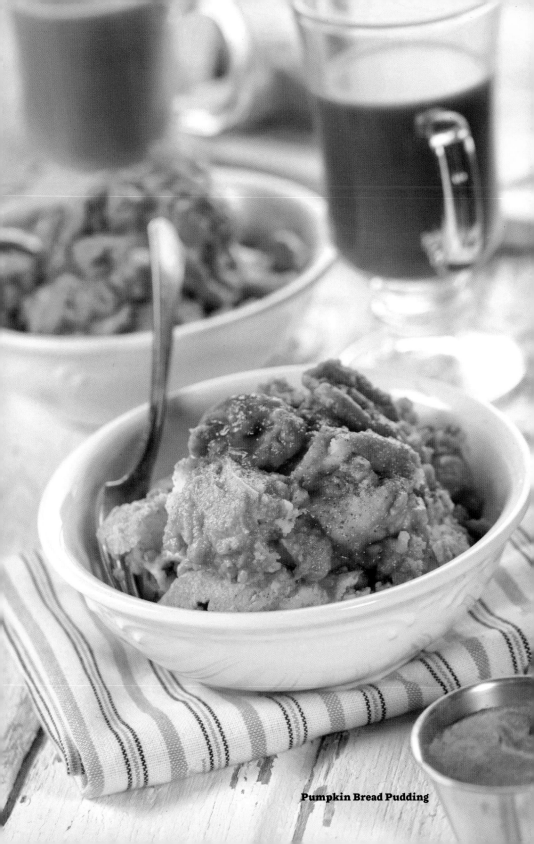

Pumpkin Bread Pudding

Barbara Burke, Newport News, VA

The Easiest Rice Pudding

We love old-fashioned rice pudding, and this version made in the slow cooker is so simple! We like to sprinkle a little bit of cinnamon and sweetened flaked coconut over ours for extra flavor.

Makes 10 servings

8 c. whole milk
1 c. long-cooking brown rice, uncooked
1/2 c. sugar
3 eggs
1/4 c. light cream
3/4 c. dried cranberries
2 t. vanilla extract
1/2 t. cinnamon
1/4 t. salt

Spray a slow cooker with non-stick vegetable spray; set aside. In a bowl, combine milk, uncooked rice and sugar; mix well. Spoon milk mixture into slow cooker. Cover and cook on low setting for 5 hours, or until rice is tender. When rice is tender, beat together eggs, cream and remaining ingredients. Whisk 1/2 cup of milk mixture from slow cooker into egg mixture. Continue whisking in the milk mixture, 1/2 cup at a time, until only half remains in slow cooker. Spoon everything back into slow cooker; stir. Cover and cook on low setting for one hour.

Nutrition Per Serving: 265 calories, 8g total fat, 4g sat fat, 23mg cholesterol, 140mg sodium, 43g carbohydrate, 1g fiber, 8g protein

★ SKINNY SECRET ★ A tiny amount of high-fat real cream goes a long way in this recipe. The whole milk lends plenty of richness, while the starch released from the rice gives this treat its smooth and velvety consistency.

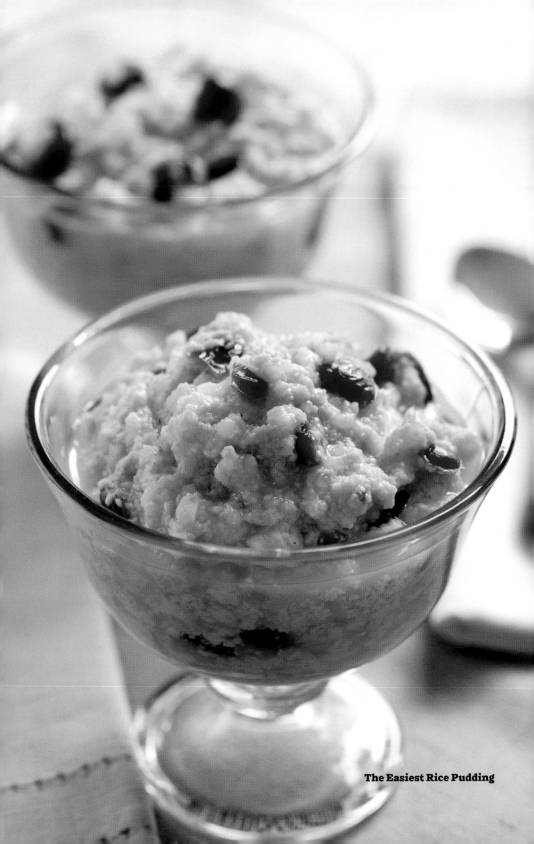

The Easiest Rice Pudding

Connie Bryant, Topeka, KS

Honeyed Apple Treat

This dessert is one my friend Ellen shared with our family when I was feeling a bit under the weather. She brought along a dozen fresh eggs from her hens as well...what a farmgirl!

Makes 8 servings

4 tart apples, peeled, cored and sliced
2 c. low-fat granola with raisins
1/4 c. honey
2 T. butter, melted
1 t. cinnamon
1/2 t. nutmeg
**Optional: whipped topping,
    additional nutmeg**

Combine apples and granola in a slow cooker. In a separate bowl, combine honey, butter, cinnamon and nutmeg; pour over apple mixture and mix well. Cover and cook on low setting for 8 hours. Garnish servings with a dollop of whipped topping and sprinkle with additional nutmeg, if desired.

Nutrition Per Serving: 202 calories, 4g total fat, 2g sat fat, 8mg cholesterol, 90mg sodium, 41g carbohydrate, 5g fiber, 4g protein

★ LOW-CAL ADD-ON ★ A one-tablespoon dollop of whipped topping will add only 10 calories to each serving.

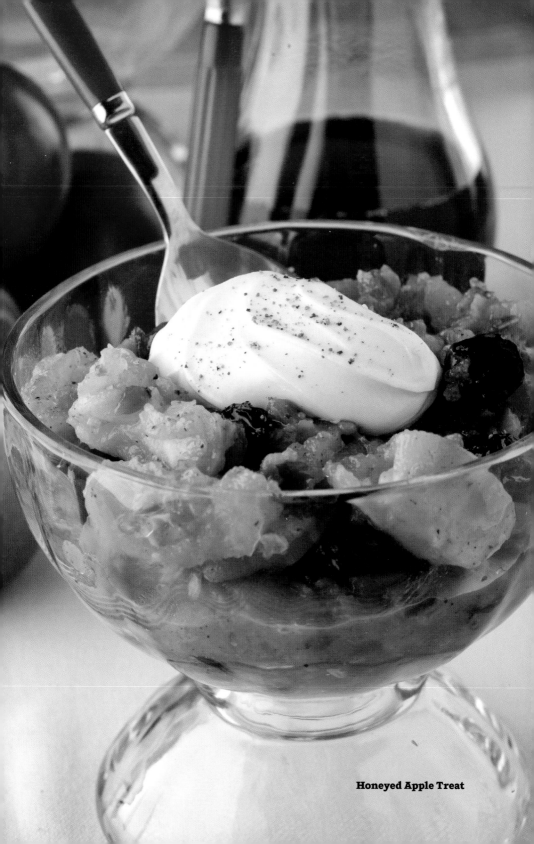

Honeyed Apple Treat

Missy Abbott, Hickory, PA

Bananas Foster

My family has loved this dessert ever since we first tried it in an upscale restaurant. We longed to taste it again...with this recipe, we can, without all the fuss and expense! To serve, spoon over scoops of ice cream.

Makes 8 servings

4 bananas, sliced
1/4 c. butter, melted
1 c. brown sugar, packed
1/3 c. spiced rum or apple juice
1 t. vanilla extract
1 t. cinnamon
1/4 c. chopped walnuts

Spray a 3-quart slow cooker with non-stick vegetable spray; layer banana slices in the bottom. In a bowl, mix together remaining ingredients; spoon over bananas. Cover and cook on low setting for 2 to 3 hours.

Nutrition Per Serving: 255 calories, 8g total fat, 4g sat fat, 15mg cholesterol, 54mg sodium, 41g carbohydrate, 2g fiber, 1g protein

Emma Brown, Saskatchewan, Canada

Lemony Pear Delight

My family loves it when early fall rolls around so we can load up on pears at the farmers' market. We usually eat them fresh, but when we want a quick & easy yet fancy dessert, this is our go-to.

Makes 8 servings

8 pears, peeled, halved and cored
1 t. lemon zest
2 T. lemon juice
1/3 c. brown sugar, packed
1/4 t. nutmeg
1/2 c. 1/3-less-fat cream cheese, softened
1/4 c. light whipping cream
3 T. chopped pecans
1/2 c. sugar cookies, crushed

In a bowl, combine pears, lemon zest and juice; toss gently to coat pears. Sprinkle brown sugar and nutmeg over pears; stir. Spoon pear mixture into a slow cooker. Cover and cook on high setting for 1-1/2 to 2 hours, until pears are soft. Spoon pears into serving bowls. Stir cream cheese and whipping cream into juices in slow cooker. Increase heat to high setting and cook, whisking occasionally, until cream cheese is melted. Evenly spoon cream cheese mixture over pears; sprinkle with pecans and crushed sugar cookies.

Nutrition Per Serving: 243 calories, 9g total fat, 4g sat fat, 20mg cholesterol, 95mg sodium, 43g carbohydrate, 6g fiber, 3g protein

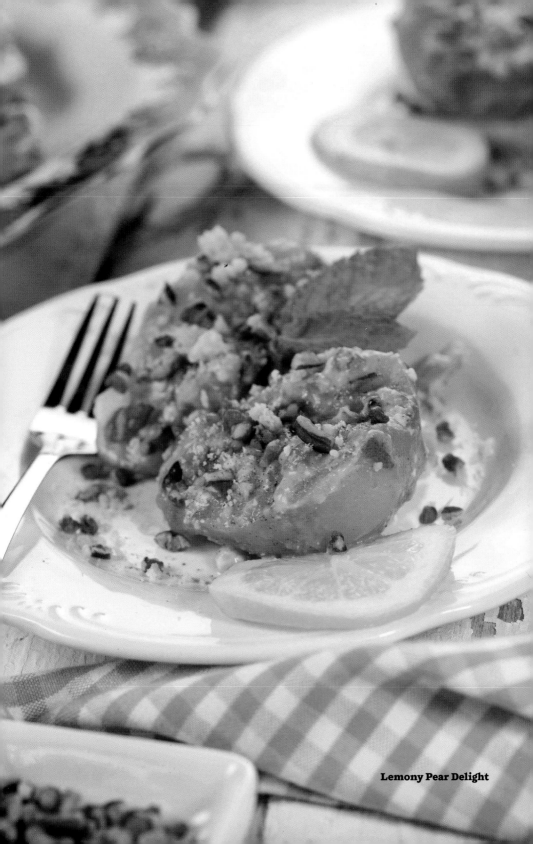

Lemony Pear Delight

Janis Parr, Ontario, Canada

Candy-Apple Tapioca

This yummy dessert is really
two delectable desserts in one...
creamy tapioca pudding and
sweet cinnamon-spiced apples!

Makes 8 servings

**8 McIntosh apples, peeled, cored and
thinly sliced**
2/3 c. sugar
1/4 c. instant tapioca, uncooked
3 T. red cinnamon candies
1/2 c. 2% reduced-fat milk
Optional: whipped cream

Place apples in a lightly greased slow
cooker. In a bowl, stir together sugar,
tapioca, candies and milk. Pour sugar
mixture over apples. Cover and cook
on high setting for 3 to 4 hours. Stir
well before serving. Top servings
with a dollop of whipped cream, if
desired.

Nutrition Per Serving: 183 calories, 1g
total fat, 0g sat fat, 1mg cholesterol, 1mg
sodium, 45g carbohydrate, 0g fiber, 1g
protein

★ LOW-CAL ADD-ON ★ For extra richness,
top this fall-spiced dessert with light vanilla
ice cream. A small 1/4-cup scoop will add only
50 calories to each serving.

Index

U. S. to Metric Recipe Equivalents

Volume Measurements

¼ teaspoon . . . . 1 mL
½ teaspoon . . . . 2 mL
1 teaspoon . . . . 5 mL
1 tablespoon = 3 teaspoons . . . . 15 mL
2 tablespoons = 1 fluid ounce . . . . 30 mL
¼ cup . . . . 60 mL
⅓ cup . . . . 75 mL
½ cup = 4 fluid ounces . . . . 125 mL
1 cup = 8 fluid ounces . . . . 250 mL
2 cups = 1 pint = 16 fluid ounces . . 500 mL
4 cups = 1 quart . . . . 1 L

Weights

1 ounce . . . . 30 g
4 ounces . . . . 120 g
8 ounces . . . . 225 g
16 ounces = 1 pound . . . . 450 g

Baking Pan Sizes

Square

8x8x2 inches . . . . 2 L = 20x20x5 cm
9x9x2 inches . . . . 2.5 L = 23x23x5 cm

Rectangular

13x9x2 inches . . . . 3.5 L = 33x23x5 cm

Loaf

9x5x3 inches . . . . 2 L = 23x13x7 cm

Round

8x1-1/2 inches . . . . 1.2 L = 20x4 cm
9x1-1/2 inches . . . . 1.5 L = 23x4 cm

Recipe Abbreviations

t. = teaspoon   ltr. = liter
T. = tablespoon   oz. = ounce
c. = cup   lb. = pound
pt. = pint   doz. = dozen
qt. = quart   pkg. = package
gal. = gallon   env. = envelope

Oven Temperatures

300° F . . . . 150° C
325° F . . . . 160° C
350° F . . . . 180° C
375° F . . . . 190° C
400° F . . . . 200° C
450° F . . . . 230° C

Kitchen Measurements

A pinch = ⅛ tablespoon
1 fluid ounce = 2 tablespoons
3 teaspoons = 1 tablespoon
4 fluid ounces = ½ cup
2 tablespoons = ⅛ cup
8 fluid ounces = 1 cup
4 tablespoons = ¼ cup
16 fluid ounces = 1 pint
8 tablespoons = ½ cup
32 fluid ounces = 1 quart
16 tablespoons = 1 cup
16 ounces net weight = 1 pound
2 cups = 1 pint
4 cups = 1 quart
4 quarts = 1 gallon